W9-AKB-133

When Sickness Heals

When Sickness Heals

THE PLACE OF RELIGIOUS BELIEF IN HEALTHCARE

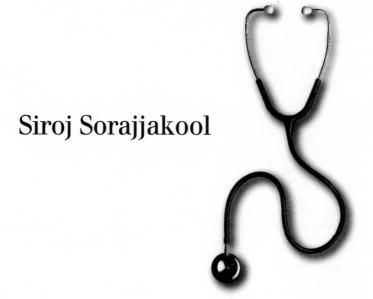

Siroj Sorajjakool

TEMPLETON FOUNDATION PRESS · PHILADELPHIA AND LONDON

Templeton Foundation Press
300 Conshohocken State Road, Suite 670
West Conshohocken, PA 19428
www.templetonpress.org

© 2006 by Siroj Sorajjakool

All rights reserved. No part of this book may be used or reproduced, stored in a retrieval system, or transmitted in any form or by any means, electronic, mechanical, photocopying, recording, or otherwise, without the written permission of Templeton Foundation Press.

Designed & typeset by Kachergis Book Design

Templeton Foundation Press helps intellectual leaders and others learn about science research on aspects of realities, invisible and intangible. Spiritual realities include unlimited love, accelerating creativity, worship, and the benefits of purpose in persons and in the cosmos.

Library of Congress Cataloging-in-Publication Data
Sorajjakool, Siroj.
    When sickness heals : the place of religious belief in healthcare /
        Siroj Sorajjakool.
            p. cm.
    Includes bibliographical references.
    ISBN-13: 978-1-59947-090-0 (pbk. : alk. paper)
    ISBN-10: 1-59947-090-X (alk. paper)
    1. Medical care—Religious aspects.   2. Spirituality.   I. Title.
    BL65.M4S67 2006
    201'.7621—dc22

                                    2005029347

Printed in the United States of America

06   07   08   09   10   10 9 8 7 6 5 4 3 2 1

To *Kathleen Greider, Christa McNerney, Gerald Winslow, Wesley Amundson,* and *Huiling Lee Sorajjakool* for contributing significantly to my growth in the world of academia

Pain and joy

I lost something of myself walking by the sea today,
The thirsty tide drags it all from the dry sand,
swallowing what is nothing and what is precious
in the same careless constancy.
Salty brine tugs everything from me, with a
regularity I never can resist.
I do not mind the sorrow
gone with the wash of water, glad at pain's farewell.
So joy and pain are forever bound inside
my paradox experience:
Pained to see my joy sliced to shreds
by grievous loss,
joyous when bright happiness
smoothes the razor edge of sorrow.

Must pain carve the well of joy?
A marriage and consummation of flint and light:
same elemental stuff, different structure as
coal and diamond are both carbon.
Both pierce and send me to new heights
of understanding this walk by the sea.

Without my scarred hand in the painful grasp of sorrow,
my heart does not rise in thankfulness for joy
and without the strong assurance of joy
the stabbing pangs of pain I cannot endure.

You knew it was
worth all pain, loss, absence
to gain all joy and wonder,
knowing too well that because
we chose death dark pain over constant felicity
it would cost you all our deep pain
to give us the wondrous joy
of knowing your heart.

—Amanda Kuhnhausen
Loma Linda University School of Medicine, Class of 2008

Contents

Acknowledgments

I wish to thank my former dean, Dr. Gerald Winslow, for encouraging me to construct a model of spiritual development within the context of healthcare that would provide practical implications for the art of spiritual care. I am very grateful to Gayle Foster for taking the time to go through the manuscript and offer insightful suggestions. Many thanks to my colleagues, Dr. Carla Gober, Dr. Johnny Ramirez, and Dr. Christy Billock, for enlightening conversations on negative theology and the role of shadows in the clinical context. I am greatly indebted to the medical students with whom I have discussed the topic of spiritual care during my past ten years of teaching at Loma Linda University. Finally, I would like to express my utmost appreciation for my wife, Huiling Lee, and my son, Chanchai, for accommodating my shadows.

Introduction

I remember as a little boy sitting on a rock by Bang Saeng beach[1] staring at my grandfather. Perhaps I was too young to understand, but I sensed that something unpleasant, very unpleasant, was haunting him. He sat on a big gray rock, watching the sun setting and staring into the ocean, lost in his own thoughts. I could see the sadness in his eyes. He was not the usual strong, vocal, and upbeat person that I knew. Except for the sound of wind and waves, he had no words. I was later told that he had lung cancer. He knew he did not have much time left. Looking back, I can't help but wonder what went through his mind.

When something out of the ordinary takes place, we have to take time out to ponder it. Tragedy disrupts the flow of time. Or perhaps tragedy acquaints us with another dimension of time and space, a space to wonder about the senselessness of tragedy, yet to discover meaning within the presence of pain.

Can there be meaning and purpose in suffering, and even in death itself? My grandfather lived in poverty for most of his hard life. Later, good fortune became a part of his reality. Upon learning that the end of his life was rapidly approaching, he was determined to build a house for us, and he personally supervised the building of it until a couple of months before he died. I do not know what went through his mind as he sat by the beach that evening. But I do know that our family would have suffered much more if he had not made that decision to provide for his children and grandchildren. What meaning did he find in the face of death?

Sickness involves more than just the body. Perhaps much more. Leo Buscaglia said it truly, "What is essential is invisible to the eye."[2] The soul is the very essence of who we are. Meaning is to our souls what air is for our bodies. Hence in sickness there is much wondering, pondering, and cogitating in each person's quest to find meaning. Is it possible for sickness to bring about a radical change of perspective on life that can result in a discovery of meaning, meaning that brings healing to the soul? Can there be meaning in much pain? Or perhaps the reverse of this question may be posited: Can there be pain without meaning?

In the following pages I set forth a theory supporting the possibility that sickness can bring about changes in existential meaning and thus offer healing to the soul. This theory explores the developmental tasks that individuals with severe illness go through in relation to the place of religion and spirituality in their experience. My ideas have grown out of ten years of teaching spiritual care to students at Loma Linda University, particularly to second-year medical students. During this time I have struggled with the literature, research, theology, students' reflections, and experiences of patients and health-care providers in the context of my efforts to conceptualize the relationship between spirituality, religion, and health, and to offer a model of spiritual care consistent with this emerging conceptualization.

I was initially interested in research on spirituality and health that indicated the numerous benefits of church attendance, prayer, meditation, scripture reading, and religious values, among others. Deciding to take a more proactive approach to the topic, Bryn Seyle, my research assistant at the time, and I decided to explore the place of spirituality among breast cancer patients. We were amazed to discover the complexity of the nature of faith and its implications for healing.

Analysis of the transcriptions of our verbatim interviews with these patients showed us that those with great faith in God's intervention actually took longer to recover emotionally, while those who saw cancer as just random reality coped better and recovered faster. This led to my renewed interest in the theological and philosophical literature that directs believers toward the role of nonbeing (referring to the negative elements in life such as illness, sorrow, misfortune, and death) in the journey of faith. I was also drawn to reflect on the meaning of religious symbols that point in this direction, such as yin and yang, labyrinth, alchemy, the goddess Kali, mandala, and others. Through this reflection, I learned that the pathway toward healing leads most often through the realm of spirituality and religion.

In this book, I first propose that spirituality is the quest for meaning. This quest is ontological in nature. It is there in a Kantian sense; it is there a priori. Similarly, the sense of transcendence is there at the ontological level as well. These two forces coexisting in one's being define the meaning of spirituality.

In support of this argument I make reference to the work of William James, based on his *Varieties of Religious Experience,* but focus primarily on the work of three individuals: the concept of myth in the writings of Raimundo Panikkar, the religious function of the psyche according to Carl Jung, and the theology of New Being from the perspective of Paul Tillich.

Second, I show that out of these two intertwining forces came religion and religious practices, including rituals and symbols. From this understanding of religion, I argue that illness leads us to question our sense of meaning. That which does not fit into our system of meaning has to be reconfigured and reintegrated. This task is developmental in nature. Numerous studies on the relationship between religion and health show positive outcomes, suggesting that the practice of religion and spirituality enhances health and nurtures one's psychological well-being.[5]

While I am positively influenced by this research, my argument takes a different turn, proposing that, even when there is no improvement in health or possibility of recovery from terminal illness, in a very important way, gaining a sense of meaning heals. In support of this developmental view I cite social science research in this area. Support from theological literature is also cited, particularly the works of Dietrich Bonhoeffer, Paul Tillich, and John Macquarrie. Besides theological literature, other religious teachings point to this integration as well, so I will cite a number of religious symbols in various religions, such as Taoism, Hinduism, and others (please reference Appendix 1 for the definitions of unfamiliar terms). Chapter six includes an attempt to apply this concept to the field of mental health, showing that a similar process occurs with those who struggle with mental illness. Taking this conceptual model into the realm of praxis, I explore this process of integration by looking at the life and writings of Søren Kierkegaard that point to the path that led him finally to come to terms with his struggle.

The last two chapters focus on implications for the practice of spiritual care by first looking at the place of spiritual assessment from the perspective of the integrative process and then exploring the practice of spiritual care based primarily on theological and religious understanding.

When Sickness Heals

CHAPTER ONE

Spirituality | Toward a Definition

At the immortal touch of thy hands my little heart loses its
limits in joy and gives birth to utterance ineffable.
Thy infinite gifts come to me only on these very small
hands of mine. Ages pass, and still thou pourest,
and still there is room to fill.

—Rabindranath Tagore, *Gitanjali*

This chapter explores the meaning and the basis of spirituality. It argues that spirituality is the ontological drive toward meaning, the need to have meaning. This need propels us toward the quest for understanding the self within this phenomenal world. Secondly, there also resides within the structure of being (and inherently within each of us) a basic sense of transcendence. Three theorists who explored spirituality from the perspective of the basic ontological drive support this understanding of spirituality. Raimundo Panikkar speaks of the existence of myth as an existential reality and its essence for the growth and development of humanity. Carl Jung proposes the concept of the religious function of the psyche. Paul Tillich puts forth the importance of the ontological drive toward New Being.

Spiritual Quest

If we had to live every day from field to meal, the narratives of our collective lives from century to century might only be about producing crops and perfecting culinary skills. Life would be plain and lacking in color. But the reality of our history is filled with traces of color and collections of art from artists who paint souls. Generations have passed, and yet our souls never cease to flourish, expressing themselves in various rhythms and forms.

This spiritual quest is captured in the poetic expression of ninth-century Irish monasticism:

> A hedge of trees surrounds me,
> A blackbird's voice sings to me;
> Above my lined book
> The call of birds chants to me.
> In a grey mantel from the topmost bush
> The cuckoo sings:
> Truly may the good Lord protect me;
> At peace I shall write under the green canopy.[1]

It is articulated by South African novelist and activist Alan Paton:

Give us courage, O Lord, to stand up and be counted, to stand up for those who cannot stand up for themselves, to stand up for ourselves when it is needful to do so. . . . Let us have no other god before thee, whether nation or party or church. Let us seek no other peace but the peace which is thine, and make us its instruments, opening our eyes and our ears and our hearts, so that we should know always what work of peace we may do for thee.[2]

And is expressed by the fourteenth-century mystic: "As the cloud of unknowing lies above you, between you and your God, you must fashion a cloud of forgetting beneath you, between you and every creature."[3]

There are numerous theories and constructs attempting to explain and define spirituality. In a Judeo-Christian upbringing, one is constantly being reminded (both positively and negatively) of the need to form a relationship with God, a relationship often defined by length of prayer and quality time spent reading the Bible.[4] Multidimensional expressions of spirituality are abundant. It is union with the divine, as in Tibetan Buddhism, unification of the self with the Atman, the making of merits, monastic contemplation, prostration of the self, the recital of sacred mantras, the nonviolence of *ahimsa*,[5] political engagement for liberation, and service to the impoverished, to name a few. Primal religions speak of a sense that there is something more than the material world in which we live. The prevailing sense of sacredness across time and culture seems to suggest something very basic in all of us. What is this something?

Spirituality and the Structure of Being

A young woman sat across from me in my office. She believed she had been fully cured from breast cancer. Others thought she was in remission. She had been through surgery, chemotherapy, and belonged to a support group for breast cancer patients. But there were questions that needed to be answered. Perhaps for this very reason, I had the opportunity to get to know her. The intake form indicated a request for a pastoral counselor, not a clinical psychologist or a marriage and family therapist. As I listened to her concerns, it became clear that she was seeking a reason for her cancer, a theological explanation. She was deeply convinced that there has to be a reason; otherwise, in her reality, it just did not make sense for someone to have to go through such a painful process both physically and psychologically. She needed a reason—a theological one, to be precise. She considered herself to be a very spiritual person. But this spiritual self-identity was a recent development, a post-diagnosis spiritual phenomenon. My client's story reflects this very need to make sense of her life.

My three-year-old nephew is famous for saying "Why, Daddy?" whenever he's asked to put things away. I suppose he thinks life is about play and work does not make any sense. In observing children, Kelly Bulkeley writes: "I've developed a deep appreciation for the powerful drive young children have to understand and make sense of the world around them. Children really, really want to figure things out—they want to know how things work, where things go, why things happen the way they do.[6]

I often wonder whether Ludwig Wittgenstein's *Tractatus*[7] may perhaps be his attempt at understanding and coming to term with his own insanity, his inability to stop thinking and pondering, and hence his need to propose that there are things one cannot talk about, a realm of mystery. Commenting on Wittgenstein's attraction to mysticism, Bertrand Russell writes:

It all started from William James's *Varieties of Religious Experience*, and grew (not unnaturally) during the winter he spent alone in Norway before the war, when he was nearly mad. Then during the war a curious thing happened. He went on duty to the town of Tarnov in Galicia, and happened to come upon a bookshop . . . he went inside and found that it contained just one book; Tolstoy on The Gospels. . . . He read it and re-read it. . . . He has penetrated deep into mystical ways of thought and feeling, but I think (though he wouldn't agree) that what he likes best in mysticism is its power to make him stop thinking.[8]

Wittgenstein's struggle reminds me of Nietzche's famous quote: "The riddle which man must solve." Perhaps this riddle is inherent in all of us. It seems that whenever we experience something that lies beyond the realm of the ordinary, we have the need to find answers and explanations, to make meaning. In *Transforming Dreams*, Bulkeley suggests that dreams represent one's attempt at understanding life's events that do not make sense. For this very reason, individuals who experienced traumatic events often have recurring dreams. "Bad dreams are attempts to make sense of bad experiences. A truly traumatic event can overwhelm a person's ordinary means of processing information; emotionally and cognitively, the experience just 'doesn't compute.'"[9] Could this urgency to make sense of one's experiences within the phenomenal world form the basis of what we have come to call "spirituality"?

I have often wondered about the meaning of spirituality. Reflecting on the history that captures the creative depths of souls confirms my intuition that spirituality is an existential quest for meaning. An archetype deeply rooted in our psyches, it expresses itself as it interacts with sociocultural, historical, and environmental contexts. Patricia Killen and John de Beer have succinctly described this process: "We are drawn to meaning. We need meaning as much as we need food and drink. Our reflection is rooted in this human drive to understand, to make the truest and richest meaning possible of our lives."[10] Or, in the words of the great mystic, Rumi:

You dance inside my chest,
  where no one sees you.
but sometimes I do, and that
  sight becomes this art.[11]

This "dance inside my chest" propels us to search for the meaning to which we belong. As we examine these variations of spiritual expressions in different faces and forms, from place to place and culture to culture, I would like to propose that this yearning is a common element inherent in humanity, the very source of spirituality itself. Spirituality is the quest to make sense of our reality and that quest is part of the structure of our being. It is both ontological and archetypal. It creates meaning, art, culture, and learning. It gives birth to science and philosophy. The richness of humanity from poetry to science, from technology to art, from philosophy to architecture, emerges from the spiritual self's need to give meaning to its reality. This reality includes the phenomenal world in which we live, the sociocultural self, and the internal-emotional self. There is a sense in which we long to know our place in the universe, our place in the culture within which we live, our place within our own subculture, and our place within ourselves.[12]

Besides the quest for meaning and the quest to make sense of oneself, there seems to exist also a transcendental element within the structure of our being. There seems to exist, within the realm of human experience, a spectrum of affects that cannot be explained rationally. But they are there, nevertheless. As Pascal puts it:

When I consider the short duration of my life, swallowed up in the eternity before and after, the little space which I fill, and even can see, engulfed in the infinite immensity of spaces of which I am ignorant, and which know me not, I am frightened, and am astonished at being here rather than there; for there is no reason why here rather than there, why now rather than then. Who has put me here? But whose order and direction have this place and time been allotted to me?[13]

To Tillich, the desire for ultimacy in the structure of being is universal. Commenting on the atheistic outlook of Hinayana Buddhism and the rise of Bodhisattva in Mahayana Buddhism, Radhakrishnan writes, "a cold, passionless metaphysics devoid of religious teaching could not long inspire enthusiasm and joy."[14] "The instinctive appetite or demand for God," states Bosanquet, "is a proof of the reality of Deity, in the same sort of sense in which hunger is a proof of the existence of food."[15] According to Paul Johnson, "It is as if there were in the human consciousness a sense of reality, a feeling of objective presence, a perception of what we may call 'something there,' more deep and more general than any of the special particular senses by which the current psychology supposes existent realities to be originally revealed."[16] In "Models and the Future of Theology," E. H. Cousin speaks of religious experience as having a dimension of depth that has no correlate in our experience of this physical universe: an experience that touches the innermost part of the person and possesses in itself a creative power that helps one see the world in a new way.[17] Speaking of religious experience, William James affirms: "I spoke of the convincingness of these feelings of reality, and I must dwell a moment longer on that point. They are as convincing to those who have them as any direct sensible experience can be, and they are, as a rule, much more convincing than results established by mere logic ever are."[18]

This brief survey is a reminder of Kant's a priori as the ground for the moral imperative. Kant argues that we are born with a certain given knowledge about reality, which makes it possible for us to interact with the world and provides us with a sense of morality. Hence, to Kant, it is the very ground that serves in the preservation of the divine reality.

A more in-depth exploration of the root of spirituality as inherent in one's ontological structure follows. We will look at the writings of three theorists: Raimundo Panikkar, Carl Jung, and Paul Tillich. (For further clarification, please see Appendix 2.)

Raimundo Panikkar

This dimension of depth and this ontological drive, according to Raimundo Panikkar, is expressed in his understanding of myth.

"Humankind," says Panikkar, "cannot live without myth."[19] The need to create narratives and tell stories is innate in humanity. Story gives meaning and adds sense to fragmented events in our lives by weaving them into a narrative with a divine calling. It turns us into players and events into plots. This, to Panikkar, makes myth an essential part of humanity. We cannot live without myth, because it is part of human experience, what Panikkar calls "that fundamental area of human experience."[20] It is a part of the fundamental human experience because myth is a form of the expression of human consciousness similar to "the central experience of Taoism, which invites us to regain the un-carved block, or of Shinto, which emphasizes an un-thought communion, an ontic solidarity with the whole of reality."[21]

Another important aspect of myth is that it transcends rationality. "Myth," says Panikkar, "is not an 'object', but an instrument of knowing, a fundamental human attitude, if you like, beside, not in front of, the logos."[22] When we make myth an object of knowledge, we destroy myth. This concept of myth reflects "inner connection" within the structure of being that transcends logic. It is intuitive.[23] Reality cannot be limited to only what we can grasp by our reasoning. Myth connects us to the reality within ourselves and to the world around us. "Myth gives us a reference point that orients us in reality."[24] Seeing myth as a form that connects us with our inner reality suggests the universal quest within humanity for the authenticity of the self. Myth is universal, and the universality of myth reflects an element within the structure of human beings seeking to direct the self toward the quintessence of being itself. Hence, myth provides a vision of the self that is integrative[25] as opposed to a vision of the self based on rationality, which may alienate self from itself. In describing the role of myth, Panikkar writes, "*Mythos* has guided me in two ways: first, it taught me to accept the *dharma* of my concrete existence (more than just choosing it); second, it taught me to dedicate myself to living a new kind of spirituality."[26]

Carl Jung

According to Carl Jung, something inherent within our psyche drives us toward religion. He calls this the religious function of the psyche. The main goal of the religious function is to drive a person toward growth and wholeness To Jung, if we were to listen carefully to our souls, we would find ourselves moving closer and closer toward wholeness, because this religious function is a driving force within our being speaking to us through various means. It appears to us through religious symbols, dreams, and the experience of the numinous. At times it can appear to us through our negative experiences. To Jung, God is always trying to speak to us through the depth of our psyche and the unconscious process. If we were to pay close attention, we would find ourselves moving toward wholeness. This movement toward wholeness is, to Jung, religious in nature. It is religious because religion's primary aim is to help people become whole. Therefore, in Jung's writings, the inner longing and yearning inherent within the structure of being is a primary source of growth. It is our very soul.

Paul Tillich

An understanding of the inner (ontological) drive toward meaning is clearly expressed in the writings of Paul Tillich and his discussion of the structure of human beings. To Tillich, human beings are constantly engaged in asking ontological questions.[27] By "ontology," Tillich means questions that naturally emerge from our inner being, questions about the existence of God and the meaning of our existence. Human beings are not who we essentially were. Because of sin, we are in a stage of estrangement from our essential nature. And because we are estranged from our essential nature, the natural process, emerging from the structure of who we are, is the quest for essential being. We look, explore, and ask questions in order to understand and to make the appropriate transition to where we ought to be. Reflecting on Tillich's ontology, John Dourley writes, "Tillich presupposes man is driven to ask the question of God because of his experience of his dialectical unity with and distance from God."[28] And while the human structure presupposes the question of God, "God," to Tillich, "is the answer to the question implied in human finitude. This answer cannot be derived from the analysis of existence,"[29] but from revelation itself.

Conclusion

This brief description of Raimundo Panikkar, Carl Jung, and Paul Tillich's approaches contains a common theme: the argument for a basic drive within the structure of being that moves toward meaning and redemption. To Panikkar, it is mythology; to Jung, the religious function of the psyche; and to Tillich, an element within the structure of being that drives human beings to move from existence to essence and from estrangement to New Being. Something within us yearns and longs for a connection, for meaning and understanding. The richness of spiritual reflections from these individuals reminds us of numerous others who have expressed similar convictions. An agnostic student once came to my office and told me that whenever he looked up into the vastness of the universe, he could not help but experience a sense of awe and wonder before something much bigger than him that comforts and consoles. St. Augustine writes, "For Thou hast made us for Thyself and our hearts are restless till they rest in Thee."[50] A sense of awe, according to Rudolf Otto, speaks to the divine connection. In the *Variety of Religious Experiences*, William James suggests, "'religions' . . . we are obliged, on account of their extraordinary influence upon action and endurance, to class them amongst the most important biological functions of mankind."[51]

After years of researching spirituality from the study of brain activities, Andrew Newberg and Eugene d'Aquili suspected that they might have discovered

evidence that the mystical experiences of our subjects—the altered states of mind they described as the absorption of the self into something larger—were not the result of emotional mistakes or simple wishful thinking, but were associated instead with a series of observable neurological events, which, while unusual, are not outside the range of normal brain function. In other words, mystical experience is biologically, observably, and scientifically real.[52]

Perhaps we can define spirituality as the coexistence of the inner realization of something bigger than ourselves and the inner ontological drive to make sense and make meaning of our existence within the physical, sociopolitical, environmental, and intrapsychic world in which we find our existence.

This leads us to the next logical question. What is the relationship between this ontological drive and the existence of religions we witness within society and our world?

CHAPTER TWO

Religion

Everything was once contained in the egg of the universe. Inside this egg slept the first living creature, P'an Ku. When P'an Ku awoke, the egg shattered. The immaculate, orderly, and light part of the egg became the sky; the unclean, heavy, and dark part became the earth. These became the forces of yin and yang. Fearing heaven and earth would weld together again, P'an Ku remained in this stance, growing ten feet a day, separating heaven and earth farther and farther apart.

P'an Ku also created the substance of things. His breath became the wind and clouds, and his voice created thunder and lightning. The sun came from his left eye, and the moon from his right eye. His arms, torso, and legs became north, south, east, west, and center. His blood became the rivers, and his veins roads and paths. From his flesh came the trees and soil. The hair on his head became the stars, and the hair on his body became the grass and flowers. His teeth and bones became metal and stone. His sweat became dew. Finally, the various parasites on his body became the first people.[1]

The aim of this chapter is to show how spirituality, as part of the structure of being, continues to describe and explain phenomena leading to the creation of myths and religions. Religious myths provide a safe space for individuals and calm the anxiety of the soul. The structuring of religion results in the creation of value systems, religious rituals, and ceremonies. To illustrate this point, I employ examples from various religious myths. These myths may appear primitive and unscientific, but we need to be cognizant of the fact that even in contemporary settings, myths abound.

Second, in the pursuit of religious truth, it is important to be aware that the role of religion is symbolic in nature. Symbol does not speak of itself, but points toward something other than itself. When it ceases to function in that way, it ceases to speak meaningfully to the current generation and, consequently, the spiritual quest moves on.

Ontology and Phenomena

In *Theology of Culture,* Tillich points out that within the structure of human reason lies the need to make meaning out of existence. Based on this need, human beings use cognitive reasoning to grasp the meaning of the ultimate in order to shape reality.[2] A scene from the movie *The Gods Must Be Crazy* is a good reminder of this inner need to explain phenomena. When a bottle dropped from the sky, a primitive man thought it must be a gift from the gods. At first, it brought pleasure and fascination, then much pain (when the children started hitting each other on the head with the bottle). Then came the theological question: Why would the gods offer a gift that brings pain? It did not make sense. So the man constructed a theological answer: The gods must be crazy.

In the previous chapter, we explored the term "spirituality" and defined it as the need to make sense of transcendence within the ontological structure. In this chapter, I argue that religion is a belief system that emerges from that inner longing for meaning. Religion is an explanation given to the phenomenal world. Religion tells stories of how things come to be and dictates ways we should respond to reality. How do we explain the origin of the earth, the moon, and the stars? What about the cycle of time and seasons, the blossoming and withering of flowers, the wind and the fire, the miracle of birth and the trauma of death? How do we explain the complexity of human behavior and emotion? How do we understand the aberrations of some and exceptional courage of others? When the world seems strange, people search for answers. Answers normalize. When the world grew dismal, the earth deities busied themselves enticing the sun goddess, Amaterasu, to come out from her hiding place in a cave.[3] When the earth was drying up, Yi came down from heaven and shot down nine suns out of ten and thus restored order over the land and sky.[4] When there was flood, there was Varaha. When there were demons, there was Narasimha.[5] With changing seasons came the story of Kung Kung:

The monster Kung Kung, having failed in an attempt to seize power from one of the Five emperors, in his fury impaled Mount Pu Chou on his horn. His attempt to destroy the world also failed, but the damage to the mountain which was the north-west pillar of the world tore a hole in the sky. In the absence of sky, the sun is unable to shine there, and instead there is a flaming dragon. This creature has a human face and a dragon's body a thousand Li in length. Its colour is red, its eyes fixed. When its eyes are open it is day; when they are closed it is night. Its exhalation is winter; its inhalation is summer. When it stops breathing there is neither rain nor wind; when it resumes breathing the wind blows. It neither eats nor drinks.[6]

Besides seeking to explain phenomena, myth helps us understand better why we do what we do. According to a peasant myth in China, people in the old days worked hard and yet did not have enough food. Often they ate every third or fourth day. This distressed the Emperor of Heaven, who decided to send the ox to convey the message that if they were to work a little harder, they would be able to eat every third day.

But the ox was stupid: he went hastily down to Earth and told men that the Emperor of Heaven had decreed that they should eat three times a day. Since the Ox had made a mistake in his instructions, he was sent back to earth to help men with their ploughing, for with only their own hands and feet it would not have been possible for men to prepare sufficient food. That is why plough-oxen, which originally were to be found only in Heaven, exist on Earth.[7]

The phenomenal world has to be interpreted and explained. The self needs to make sense of itself and cannot do so without constructs. In Christianity, we have been told about the genesis of the world. Genesis 1:1 tells us, "In the beginning God created the heavens and the earth." Then, pain occurred because of disobedience. I once heard a Chinese version of the creation story. If Eve were Chinese, sin would not have entered the world. Instead of the apple, she would have eaten the snake. That is one possible explanation. Just recently, I heard another interesting feminist version. After seven days of creation, Adam was all alone. So God told Adam God would create a woman as a partner and a friend. She would cook and clean. She would do everything to please him. She would not complain. She would take every order from him without any question. Intrigued by such a possibility, Adam asked, "What will this cost?" "An arm and a leg," God replied. "How about just a rib?" Adam inquired. The rest is history. We need explanations and there is, possibly, a lot of truth in humor.

We create myths. We tell stories. We construct and seek explanations. It is our way of making sense of our lives, of ourselves and who we are. When there is no story, life does not make sense. The truth about myth is expressed in the following poetry:

> I will tell you something about stories,
>> [he said]
> They aren't just entertainment.
>> Don't be fooled.
> They are all we have, you see,
>> all we have to fight off
>>> illness and death.
> You don't have anything
>> if you don't have the stories.
>>> Their evil is mighty
> but it can't stand up to our stories.
> so they try to destroy the stories
> let the stories be confused or forgotten.
>> They would like that
>> They would be happy
> Because we would be defenseless then.[8]

The Function of Myth

Human neurological structure exists for the purpose of human growth and survival. And myth is one of the essential tools the mind carefully constructs in order to sustain and preserve life. According to Newberg, d'Aquili, and Rause, when a person senses danger, their primary response is a heightened emotional state, creating a sense of discomfort and imbalance. A person in a state of arousal attempts to restore balance. Once the task is completed, the person returns to his or her prior state. Cognition is then activated. The riddle has to be resolved, the question must be answered, and the mystery known.

Uncertainty at such an urgent moment is intolerable to the causal operator, so it does what it is designed to do in the absence of a specific cause: it proposes one. This proposal arises out of activity in the hippocampus, the limbic structure where past experiences are stored as memories. Rapidly, the mind scours these memory banks, sorting and cross-referencing information as it searches for any pertinent content-images, sounds, or larger chunks of experience—that might shed light on the problem at hand.[9]

The creation of myth paints stories to restore the soul from anxiety. It reduces the arousal state and brings back a sense of normality. Danger is contained because within the myth we come to know its cause and hence its resolution.[10] When the pain of hunger creates the myth of drought, the primitives know which god to approach and which dance to perform. The beginning of myth, writes Newberg, d'Aquili, and Rouse, is that urgent, "unanswerable question."[11]

Once one knows the cause, one can offer the prescription. Proposing theories of drought, thunder, sickness, and death does not remove the anxiety. To calm the soul, further steps need to be taken. How can one induce Amaterasu (the sun goddess) from hiding in a cave or prevent the kitchen god from reporting mischievous happenings to heaven? And how can fishermen invoke the help of Varuna so their ship will be guided through the night in the vast ocean?

I once rented out my house in Thailand to a group of college students. One day, while trying to collect the rent, one of the students inquired if I had asked permission to inhabit that house. I was puzzled. Should not the person who owns the house have the right to inhabit it? They disagreed with me and by describing the events taking place in my house, helped me understand what they were talking about. "We saw the body of a stranger walking around in this house late at night." "It was not pleasant," they all confirmed. "Especially the sight." They asked if I could perform a ceremony to gain permission from the "stranger" to reside in my house. I told them that I could not do so because of my religion. A month later, when I came to collect the rent, I noticed a couple of joss sticks with bowls of rice and fruit in my back yard. A month later, they all moved out. Perhaps, in their minds, the stranger did not like rice and fruit. The moral of the story is that you have to know the cause of the problem and perform the right rituals. If we do not follow through with the appropriate steps, then our constructs do not mean much. There is more to myth than stories; they must be supported by lifestyle.

Beliefs and Practices

This section illustrates the emergence of religious rituals and practices from belief systems. We see numerous examples in our day-to-day living and weekly religious engagements. In Christianity, we tithe because we believe in acknowledging that all belongs to God; we take communion because we want to be a part of the death and resurrection of Christ; we practice temperance because our bodies are God's temple. Muslims pray in the name of Allah because they believe there is only one God. The first pillar of Islam, Shahada, states, "There is no God but Allah." The following three examples may seem foreign to us, but they are common practices in some parts of the world.

Thai Animism

Thai animism is a good place to start exploring the relationship between beliefs and practice. In Thai animism, there are two forms of spirits: domesticated and non-domesticated. The difference between the two is predictability and unpredictability. Domesticated spirits are predictable. They respond to the right rituals and ceremonies. Non-domesticated spirits, on the other hand, are not predictable. It is a common belief that the spirits reside everywhere. For this reason, you will find a spirit-house in many homes. But there is also a town spirit, a city spirit, and a temple spirit. For travelers, the only spirit that matters is the spirit presiding over their current location: "It is not very practical or politic for a traveler to remain devoted to the guardian spirit of his village when he is away. As soon as he steps outside his village boundaries he has entered into the realm of another local ruler that he had better respect and worship."[12]

It is important to know the preferences of the particular spirit one is honoring. Evoking the spirit and searching for fulfillment of one's wishes requires appropriate rituals and an understanding of how that spirit works.

In order to invoke its benevolent attention and to activate its protection the worshipper has to initiate the action by paying respect and making a small offering. The worshipper then offers his terms of contract: if the *saksit*[13] power will fulfill his wishes, he will come back and offer a feast, a head of pig, flowers, or a theatrical performance. Most of these powers have known tastes and dislikes: The Buddha image *Pra Chinaraad* in Pitsanuloke likes pig heads, *Pra Kae. W. Morakot* (The Emerald Buddha) loves hard boiled eggs, the spirit of the *lak-myang* (city pillar) in Bangkok is fond of *lakhon chaatrii* performances, and the four-faced Brahma at the Erawan Hotel appreciates flower garlands, elephants, and a donation to the Erawan hospital foundation; female spirits (*caw-mae*) have a marked taste for phalli.[14]

Non-domesticated spirits, on the other hand, are unpredictable. They are known to live in cemeteries and forests. They may strike without being provoked and do not respond to ceremonies or rituals. The way to handle them is through the use of powerful white magic symbols based on moral goodness. Benevolent and magical monks, through their merits, may produce powerful amulets, tattoos, or formulae that can protect individuals from evil spirits.[15]

Hungry Ghosts

To many Chinese, the seventh month of the lunar calendar is the most inauspicious month, because they believe that during this month the spirits of the dead are relieved from hell to wander the earth among people. Some Chinese will not travel, marry, swim, or engage in any activity that appears risky during this time, for fear that these wandering spirits may bring harm. The origin of this belief is unknown, but believers think that the ghosts are hungry and violent because their family members did not make ritualistic offerings to them, or because they died a tragic death and are out for vengeance. Hungry ghosts make trouble for people and have an insatiable appetite for food. It is not uncommon for some Chinese associations to perform ceremonies for these hungry ghosts, whom they believe have been ignored by their families. During these ceremonies, they burn joss sticks, candles, and hell banknotes, as well as slaughter animals as offerings to appease these very hungry spirits.[16]

The Earth

Earth, according to the Ashanti and other Akan peoples, is associated with conception and vegetation. To them, the goddess Asase Ya is the goddess of fertility and vegetation. Describing the importance of Asase Ya in the lives of the Ashanti and Akan people, Roger Schmidt writes:

Sacrifices to her are made at plowing and harvesting times, and on Thursdays, her sacred day, farming is forbidden. Cultivators were not alone in deifying the earth. Remarks voiced by Smodalla, a leader of the Sahapatin tribe in the 1880s in the state of Washington, to an Indian agent trying to persuade his people to farm reflect both a mystical identification with the earth and a hunter's aversion to farming: "You ask me to plow the ground. Shall I take a knife and tear my mother's bosom? Then when I die she will not take me to her bosom to rest."[17]

Religious Implications

This recounting of the rituals and practices of animism offers an insight into the formation of religious beliefs that result in rituals and practices based on a particular worldview. In some ways, myths and rituals are ways through which human beings attempt to discover the meaning of self, which lies beyond the realm of the ordinary and reaches out toward the realm of transcendence. "Our rituals," according to Newberg, d'Aquili, and Rause, "are about something; they tell stories, and these stories give them meaning and power." They further point out, "[T]he root of the ceremonial rites of all human societies, from the most primitive to the most exalted, are an elaboration of the neurobiological need of all living things to escape the limiting boundaries of the self."[18]

Hence, we may be able to say that religion has its root in the inner desire to make sense of the phenomenal world (external reality and internal psyche). As a belief system becomes more complex and systematic, a value system emerges based on the newly acquired worldview. Value systems result in religious practices and rituals, thus completing the cycle of the need to explain and understand as a way of making sense of one's reality.

Limits of Religion

Religion, as a construct that attempts to make meaning in relation to transcendence, needs to remain true to this transcendental pole within the ontological structure itself. Through various constructs, religion upholds and nurtures human spirits through difficult times by offering meanings that are unavailable through other means. It sustains and offers a resting place for weary souls. One knows that there is something out there bigger than we are, designing, reconfiguring, and choreographing lives and human history. But there is a limit to our sense of certainty, because the rest lies within the mysteries of life, God, and the universe. The greater challenge is to recognize that we are a part of this mystery and unfolding reality. There is a sense, as we grow up in this culture, to think that we are not a part of objective reality, that it stands outside of us as an object we must possess (whether it be in terms of knowledge or physical manipulation). And this sense applies to our attitude toward God as well.

We think we are constantly moving toward a better understanding of this objectivity. There is greater proximity. We know more and perhaps soon may congratulate ourselves for possessing knowledge of this absolute reality. We try, and the more we try, we discover emerging patterns and new variables. Like a cat chasing its tail and a child chasing his or her shadow, the constant movement does not end until we realize that we are indeed a part of this reality. We participate in it. We modify, we change, we improve, and we destroy. No reality stands outside us. We are in reality, changing and being changed by it. The religious commitment is the determination to totally embrace reality and make a better society, a safer community, a more compassionate humanity, and better citizens.

But our insatiable desire for certainty betrays the core essence of our needs. We absolutize religion and normalize rituals. We form creeds and sacraments. We create aberration and polarization. We define "us" and "them." We try to win "them" over, or identify "them" as "the other." We fight, murder, and shed blood in the name of the sacred, claiming absolute knowledge of its reality. Many claims have been made and many lives sacrificed.

Perhaps the only absolute we can lay claim to is awareness of the transcendence within the structure of our beings. And, in a sense, the transcendence that finds no explanation within the everyday configuration points to something bigger and to hope for meaning in a world of chaos. And this is what we know. We attempt various constructs. Different religions give them many names. We deduce a value system and offer prescriptions for the soul. These various religions provide sustenance for their believers. But we need to be aware that, in the final analysis, God remains a mystery to us all. God is not controlled by our constructs. God does what God does. God chooses what God chooses. God just is, in a way incomprehensible to us. God said, "I Am." Religion, therefore, needs to recognize its role as a symbol of the sacred. A symbol always points to something greater than itself. It is not absolute. It only represents. It points. It cannot claim certainty in itself. Religion symbolizes. In Tillich's words, "every symbol points beyond itself to a reality for which it stands."[19]

The Problem of Our Generation

Perhaps one of the main reasons we are not able to embrace religion at a symbolic level is because we have inherited a linear thinking process that claims rationality and causal relation as proper and appropriate methods of thinking. We analyze and categorize. We create a taxonomy of reality and convince ourselves that the one who knows controls. We have become masters of navigating reality, both external and internal. But, as Jung has pointed out in *The Undiscovered Self*, the goddess of reason has only created a vacuum in the soul. Reason alienates. Through categories of right and wrong, good and bad, beautiful and ugly, righteous and sinful, smart and foolish, speech and silence, rationality ensures the preference of one over the other. But the soul is the totality of itself. It possesses all. It is both smart and foolish, right and wrong, beautiful and ugly. "Both" as a concept does not exist in rational thought.

When totality cannot be embraced, delineation takes place. Delineation results in alienation. The emergence of the postmodern is perhaps the call of the psyche for a healing of its brokenness. But one must pay attention, since the psyche will only strive for a balance. Nevertheless, that natural tendency to restore the alienated self encourages us to recognize the need to remember that life is much bigger than the mind can conceive. And so it is with reality. We are again reminded of the symbolic nature of religion. Religion symbolizes and represents. It always points beyond itself. For this very reason, spirituality continues to flourish. When religion ceases to speak meaningfully to a point in time and history because it refuses to represent and it claims absolute certainty, spirituality propels us to move on in the quest to make sense of who we are within the current sociopolitical, economic, and historical context where we find ourselves. While reexamining his faith, John Shelby Spong stated:

But do those symbols, literalized or not, still translate in this generation? Can they still convey meaning in a postmodern generation? The magic of breaking the power of death by placing blood on the doorposts or on the cross is strangely primitive. The cannibalistic ritual of eating the flesh of the deceased deity is filled with ancient psychological nuances that are disturbing to modern sensitivities.[20]

This need to question and make sense is clearly stated by Spong:

I do not believe in a deity who can help a nation win a war, intervene to cure a loved one's sickness, allow a particular athletic team to defeat its opponent, or affect the weather for anyone's benefit. I do not think it is appropriate for me to pretend that those things are possible when everything I know about the natural order of the world I inhabit proclaims that they are not.[21]

When what we were taught is incongruent with our experiences, we move on. We have to, because we are unable to live in a senseless world. Hence, spirituality is reactivated when religion ceases to serve as a symbol of transcendence and claims absoluteness without the ability to speak meaningfully to the experience of believers.

CHAPTER THREE

Illness, Meaning, and Miracles

Birth is suffering, old age is suffering, sickness is suffering, death is suffering. Involvement with what is unpleasant is suffering. Separation from what is pleasant is suffering. Also, not getting what one wants and strives for is suffering. And form is suffering, feeling is suffering, perception is suffering, karmic constituents are suffering, consciousness is suffering; in sum these five agglomerations, which are the basis of clinging to existence, are suffering. This, monks, is the Noble Truth of suffering.

—Gautama Buddha, The Teachings of Buddha as
Recorded in Tripitaka

This chapter brings our discussion on spirituality and religion into a clinical context. How does this interpretation of spirituality (as a quest for meaning) enhance our understanding of patients' struggles with illness? What happens when a person becomes seriously ill? Where is spirituality? I propose that illness and suffering play an important role in the quest for meaning. Suffering in itself does not seem to make sense. The spiritual task is to try to make sense of it. One of the initial responses of a person confronted with severe sickness or terminal illness is to turn to divine intervention to maintain his or her prior perspective on reality. This may be viewed as a necessary attempt to hold on to a sense of meaning.

A Narrative

I met Phoom in the winter of 2003 when he came to visit his sister in California. He was fifteen at that time. He was smart and energetic. His sister, Gan, stayed with our family as an exchange student for six months. My wife and I learned to love this family like our own. We kind of adopted Gan as our daughter. When I went to Thailand, I had the opportunity to see Phoom again. He had just broken his leg and was told not to play soccer. Somehow, he snuck behind his parents' backs and played soccer with crutches. A couple of months later I learned that Phoom had been diagnosed with germ cell cancer. According to his physician, he was among the few who did not respond well to treatment. I called his mother one evening, and she was at the temple. It was time for the family to make merits (good deeds) in the hope that these merit-making rituals would extend Phoom's life and provide a cure. His mother strongly believed in religious rituals. The family visited the temple frequently. Phoom himself even stayed in the temple as a novice monk for a time, practicing *dharma* and performing rituals. But it was not just because her son was sick that she performed merits. Her family had always been committed to helping charitable organizations, raising money for various temples and donating money for many good projects. In her estimate, it would be reasonable that when she needed the gods, they would be there to help her through this darkest time. A few months later, we heard the sad news that Phoom had passed away. He had begged his parents to let him go. "I'm very tired," said the seventeen-year-old. "Please let me go." It was one of the hardest chapters in their lives. It did not make much sense. His mother's religious world informed her that good deeds beget good results. The religious rituals she performed were ways of expressing religious commitment. She did much more than her share. But the gods did not heal in the presence of accumulated merits. What went wrong? Phoom's mother became discouraged and does not go to the temple as frequently as she once did.

Her religion was once her way of conceptualizing reality and it dictated her ritual practices. In the presence of incongruence, how can she make sense of this experience?

Meaning and Suffering

In *Patterns of Religion,* Roger Schmidt suggests:

Meaning giving involves more than stories of how things came to be, such as the Greek myth that fire was a gift of Prometheus, and the biblical myth that different languages came from God's confusion of tongues at the Tower of Babel. Sociologist Max Weber (1864–1920) saw religion as a way of investing life with meaning in response to those features of human existence, suffering, evil, and death that are not resolvable in scientific terms. As anthropologist Clifford Geertz observed, religious symbol systems provide a context for making suffering "bearable, supportable, something, as we say sufferable."[1]

Having taught spiritual care to medical students for the past ten years, I know that a common remark in response to addressing patients' spiritual needs is the fear of bringing up something irrelevant to patients or imposing theological/spiritual conversations that may seem inappropriate to the medical profession. I often tell students that a lot of theological reflection goes on in hospitals, hospices, rehabilitation centers, and so forth. Perhaps more is happening theologically in these locations than in seminaries. It may be less systematic, but it is certainly more existential and more intense. The reason is that often, prior to traumatic events in life, we normally define meaning in relation to that which is positive, that which is normative. Traumatic events question this definition of meaning.

Figure 1

MEANING	LACK OF MEANING
Positive, Normative	Negative, Non-normative

I remember with much clarity the often-repeated phrase that went through my mind when I was going through a major episode of depression (not realizing what it was at the time because of my lack of exposure and knowledge). In the midst of such intense mental agony (heavy clouds of darkness permeating every thought and dream), which began pushing me almost to the verge of insanity, came a repeated phrase, "There had better be something good come out of this." Life is unbearable when there is no meaning, no purpose, and no benefit from senseless suffering. It seems our psyches lack the ability to tolerate meaningless and, therefore, we are forced to believe that pain and suffering are of some benefit. What sense can we make of suffering? What sense can we make of terminal illness? What sense can we make of chronic pain?

Sheldon Cashdan told a story about a boy name Roy who was assigned to him while he was a psychologist intern at a psychiatric facility. Roy's dad was an alcoholic and his mom a prostitute who left him when he was young. At the age of three, his dad took off and left the boy locked in the house. Three days later the neighbors called the police, who came and found Roy in the middle of the kitchen eating pieces of plaster out of hunger. The boy went from one foster home to another, but no one was able to keep him because of his obsession for consuming inedibles. He was later diagnosed with pica. Through the course of therapy, the boy was getting better until, one day, as Cashdan was stepping into the session, he found Roy facing the blackboard appearing perplexed. In Cashdan's words:

The scene that greeted me was heartrending. For a split second, I didn't recognize Roy. Looking forlorn and bewildered, he had ground the chalk into a fine white powder and smeared it all over his face. He looked like a small white ghost. There were tears streaming down his face, and brown streaks showed beneath the white where the tears had washed away the chalk. Standing alone in the corner, he was a pitiful sight.

I went to Roy and held him in my arms until he stopped crying. After a while, he told me what had happened. He apparently had been spending a lot of time trying to figure out why his parents had left him. He had given a lot of thought to it and in the process had become confused and depressed. In an effort to make sense of his jumbled thoughts and jumbled feelings, he reasoned that it must have been because he was black.[2]

Most of the other children at the facility were white and they all still had their parents. Roy figured to be black was to be bad. Roy's story reflects that deep yearning to understand, especially when things go wrong in one's life. Why abandonment? Why suffering?

This very question initiated the quest in Gautama Buddha. Why pain? Why old age? Why death? Life does not seem to make sense in the face of suffering and death, and he had to find the answer to this riddle of life, to make sense of the senselessness. The quest ceased when he finally found the Four Noble Truths. Life is suffering. To be is to suffer. We suffer because we have desire. We have *tanha*.[5] When we want what we do not have, we suffer. When we have what we do not want, we suffer. If we do not want "to have" or "not to have," we will not suffer. Buddha's wisdom is profound. The less we want, the less we suffer. Therefore, the way out of suffering is to cease having desire. Cease the wants. Cessation of wants comes by practicing the Eight Noble Paths. This is the way of the Buddha, a way of making sense of suffering and death. To be is to suffer; therefore; life is that movement from being to nonbeing. But to "non-be" is a complicated process, because the Buddhist cosmology presupposes a cycle of birth and rebirth. We cannot stop the pain because we cling to life. Clinging to life leads to rebirth and rebirth to suffering. The cycle stops only when the desire "to be" and any illusion of the reality of the self ceases. Only then can one achieve nonbeing and exit the cycle of suffering.

Pain is a driving force that explains the phenomenal world in which we live. Complex systems of explanation emerge through the senselessness of pain. Pain is an active ingredient in spirituality. It creates systems, philosophy, poetry, symphony, symbols, art, and design.

> What unnumbered griefs we carry
> in our numbed hearts—
> unuttered sigh, the whispers
> of songless sparrows.
>
> "The deeper the sorrow
> the less tongue we have,"
> the *Talmud* says.
>
> Tongue-tied, heart-stung, our deepest griefs
> bury themselves alive
> in the tombs of our former selves.
> Only the welcome lament liberates them.

Let my words be to you
like the green earth cherishing.
Let this song sew up
the tattered seams of your soul.

And know, as you bathe
the body of your beloved
with bowls of rain water,
you wash her
with the very tears of God.[4]

I once met a woman during group therapy in a lock-down unit of a psychiatric facility. I was leading a group, and the young lady patiently waited to say something to the group. Finally, she spoke: "I'm not a human being." I was not completely surprised. She asked to speak to me with a sense of urgency. Right after the group session, I met with her. She informed me that she had shocking news to share. She was going to die on a certain day. I asked why and learned that she saw death as liberation from pain. This patient had moved from one foster home to another. "I never felt like I belonged, anywhere I went," she told me. "And there's always this accompanying sense of sadness." She began to construct her explanatory style one night when, in a dream, she saw herself as a wolf howling in the clouds. The dream repeated itself a number of times. She could not make sense of it. A number of years later, her dreams had a similar theme with more detail. She dreamed she was a little pup playing with her other siblings. Her parents always told her to not stray and to stay with the pack. Out of curiosity one day, she left in search of adventure. She followed a noise into the forest and was instantly killed by a wild animal. "At the very moment I was killed, my spirit went into my father's sperm. This is how I've become a human being."

I looked at her chart and learned she had been diagnosed with schizoaffective disorder. The diagnosis explained her intense sadness but not her theory of incarnation. Her belief that her true self was a wolf, an idea that fits the Hindu/Buddhist cosmology, reflected her desire to make sense of her pain and suffering, her struggle with sadness, and inability to get along with others. "I never felt I belonged." I glanced through her collection of photographs of wolves and realized the power of spirituality: her need to create an explanatory myth to sustain herself and possibly make sense of her melancholia. Becoming a human being had been the punishment for her disobedience. Thus, her suffering. Her task was to return to her original state as a wolf.

To accept her humanity she would have had to accept the senselessness of her unbearable sadness and isolation. To accept her humanity would be to accept her madness in accordance with the diagnostic criteria. To her, the unbearable sorrow of her life had to be more than merely insanity resulting from a chemical imbalance. To have madness with no meaning attached can be more unbearable than madness itself.

Suffering can have a similar effect on individuals with chronic or terminal illness. A breast cancer patient recalls her experience when she was first told she had cancer: "When the word cancer hits you, when they pronounce cancer . . . that word had a big impact. First when I heard that I just denied. More than 100% . . . one thing that I realized—I never questioned God, why me? That's the thing . . . I count my blessings, I never questioned God. But just denied it, it cannot be me. But when you hear that, how can you cope with it? . . . all you do is just deny and be angry."[5]

What sense does it make for someone who has been practicing healthful living to be told that she has breast cancer? What sense is there in pain and suffering? What sense is there in death?

David had just been informed that his cancer was at stage four. What sense did it make? Prior to the diagnosis, David had just been through a conversion experience and had wondered what God wanted him to do. Upon hearing his diagnosis, David knew his calling would be to use his experience to minister to people going through similar illnesses. He felt that something good had to come out of his experience.

While walking through the sacredness of many lives as a chaplain in an oncology unit, a common phrase I heard was: "I don't know why I have to go through this. But I believe there must be a purpose in it. I just haven't figured that out yet."

A nurse with kidney failure, staring into the face of her mortality, once said to me, "There must be a reason. I'm still trying to figure out my calling in life." In essence, she was saying, "If I have to go through so much pain and suffering and face mortality at such a young age, there's got to be a reason, a good reason." The alternative is just inconceivable. It does not come as a surprise that, after interviewing fifteen individuals with terminal illnesses, Patricia Fryback and Bonita Reinert wrote: "Finding meaning is particularly important when a person is facing a serious illness, because the illness itself causes permanent changes in life that force a re-evaluation of any previously assumed meaning."[6]

In summary, we can say that often meaning is defined as that which is positive and normative. When someone faces a trauma, the trauma causes the person to question his or her sense of meaning because in a person's usual belief system there is no meaning in trauma. And if there is no meaning in trauma, the presence of trauma suggests the lack of meaning in one's life. Often this becomes more intolerable than pain itself, since the need for meaning is ontological, and one is unable to live without meaning. Hence, people who face trauma for the first time often yearn for miracles.

Miracles

When many individuals first encounter trauma, they strongly desire divine intervention. Miracles return everything to normal. Miracles normalize life. Miracles restore meaning. When trauma causes people to question their sense of meaning, they may believe that the best thing would be for God to remove the trauma so that they can regain a sense of meaning. The traumatized person might think or say, "If God heals me, I can return to a cancer-free life because I really cannot deal with this right now." He or she invokes the Supreme Being. When my dad was told he had cancer, he became really sad and depressed. A couple of days after he learned of his diagnosis, he called the family together. He referred us to the passage in the book of Genesis about the story of Jacob before he met with his brother, Esau.

> So Jacob was left alone, and a man wrestled with him till daybreak. When the man saw the he could not overpower him, he touched the socket of Jacob's hip so that his hip was wrenched as he wrestled with the man. Then the man said, "Let me go, for it is daybreak."
>
> But Jacob replied, "I will not let you go unless you bless me."
>
> The man asked him, "What is your name?"

"Jacob," he answered.

Then the man said, "Your name will no longer be Jacob, but Israel, because you have struggled with God and with men and have overcome."[7]

Then he turned to us and said, "I'm not asking you to pray that God's will be done. I ask you to struggle with God. Just like Jacob did. Never let go. Struggle until God answers our prayer. Never let go."

Based on our previous discussion on the role of meaning and spirituality, this initial intense longing for divine intervention may be viewed as a struggle to maintain a sense of meaning based on a person's prior schema at the existential level, the schema that defines meaning by excluding negative elements. In a sense, the traumatized person is unable to make any sense of this new reality, this pain, this suffering, and this premature encounter with mortality. Meaning is still attached to life prior to the diagnosis. Cancer, kidney failure, or AIDS just do not fit into the schema. A miracle seems to be the only answer for such a detrimental diagnosis. Through miraculous intervention, cancerous cells should be magically removed so that the person will be able to maintain his or her previous system of meaning, one that does not include negative elements. Asking for divine intervention is begging to return to a previously held belief system to sustain a sense of meaning.

Belief in miraculous intervention plays a very significant role in the spiritual transformation of patients. It sustains them and provides a sense of safety. There is something truly comforting in believing that there is Someone who is much bigger, who is all-knowing, and who cares. This belief makes it possible for individuals to disengage from their anxious obsession with the overwhelming events. Belief in divine intervention also makes it possible for a person to hold on to a sense of meaning based on his or her current belief system.

Contrary to the popular belief that caregivers need to help patients face reality and thereby break the denial system, their initial denial should be treated with respect. Denial is an important defense mechanism, much like the immune system. It protects us and sustains us. Kubler-Ross's advice is for us to journey with the sick and dying even into denial, to go where they want to go and to be where they want to be. There can be a deep sense of reality in fantasy. There is much truth to be learned when a dying patient plans her wedding or when a paraplegic discusses a time in the future when he'll go surfing. Fantasy is sacred and should be treated as such. It connects us to the basic instinctive root of our being and, in a sense, forms an integral part of our souls.

I need to clarify here that believing in miracles is not equivalent to being in denial. God is God. God chooses to do what God chooses to do. And if God is God, miracles are therefore not beyond what God can do. The hard part is for us to leave this to God and let God be God.

Conclusion

In the face of trauma, people often turn to God for miraculous intervention because, by so doing, they may be able to maintain a sense of meaning by holding on to their prior belief systems. A miracle can potentially remove a deadly diagnosis and, when cancer is magically removed, a person can hold on to his or her system of meaning (life is meaningful without pain, suffering, and death). What is critical here may be the lack of meaning and not the diagnosis or the trauma itself, because the belief system is unable to offer meaning in the presence of trauma. What is intolerable is the lack of meaning more than pain itself. Under this circumstance, miraculous intervention may be the only hope for meaning.

When miracles do not take place, an individual's spiritual self calls for an integration of this "negativity" or "nonbeing," thus creating a new system of meaning, a reconfiguration that takes into consideration mortality, pain, and suffering. This developmental task will be the focus of the next chapter.

CHAPTER FOUR

Illness and the Developmental Task

It is the pang of separation that spreads throughout the world and gives birth to shapes innumerable in the infinite sky.

It is this sorrow of separation that gazes in silence all night from star to star and becomes lyric among rustling leaves in rainy darkness of July.

It is this overspreading pain that deepens into loves and desires, into sufferings and joys in human homes; and this it is that ever melts and flows in songs through my poet's heart.

—Rabindranath Tagore[1]

This chapter looks at a developmental task patients often have to go through, proposing that the essential step for traumatized patients is to make the transition from an existential desire for the removal of pain and suffering to integrating them into a system of meaning. To maintain a sense of meaning is to find ways to keep a sense of meaning in the midst of suffering itself, rather than without it. This process of integration takes place at the theological level as well.

Developmental Task

"We reflect," writes Patricia O'Connell Killen and John de Beer, "when something happens to us that we cannot readily fit into the interpretive categories we normally use to make meaning in our lives."[2] One evening my wife called me from home. She had just returned from a store with our teenage son, who was usually demanding and didn't talk to us nicely. There was deep concern in her voice as she described what happened. "I took our son to the shop and I really do not know what happened. He spoke like a normal person. He wasn't rude. He was not shouting. He was actually very nice. I just do not understand." She was trying hard to understand this unusual phenomenon of him being cordial. When something happens out of the ordinary, there is a deep yearning within us to understand it.

A Thai friend once told me how perplexed she was when she could not understand her own behavior. "When my anxiety was high," she reflected, "I just had to throw up. It would release my anxiety. I could not understand myself and neither could I stop this practice." Her journey took her to a number of professionals, but was initiated by her inner longing for self-understanding; eventually, she became aware of the impact childhood abuse had on her life.

When one's belief system is no longer able to provide meaning in the face of severe illness or major loss, spirituality is activated to perform its task. In the last chapter, I pointed out that when a person faces a critical diagnosis, he or she may seek miraculous intervention. However, when miracles do not take place, and cancer remains, the task is to reconfigure one's schema, one's sense of reality and belief system to accommodate this new devastating variable. One must integrate this new variable by modifying or expanding the existing system—by reconfiguring it. This task is essential in making meaning possible within the situation. "How can my life be meaningful when I am dying?" "How can there be purpose when I suffer constantly from excruciating pain?" To answer this type of question is to begin the task of integrating negative elements or "nonbeing" into one's system of meaning.

Figure 2

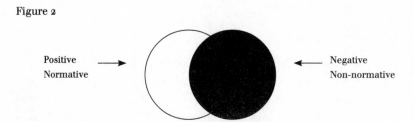

In referring to people's experiences with trauma, Judith Lewis Herman writes:

The psychiatrist Mardi Horowitz postulates a "completion principle" which "summarizes the human mind's intrinsic ability to process new information in order to bring up to date the inner schemata of the self and the world." Trauma, by definition, shatters these "inner schemata." Horowitz suggests that unassimilated traumatic experiences are stored in a special kind of "active memory," which has an "intrinsic tendency to repeat the representation of contents." The trauma is resolved only when the survivor develops a new mental "schema" for understanding what has happened.[3]

In the words of Naomi Remen:

The language of the soul is meaning. We may first discover the soul when life events awaken in us the need for meaning. In serious or chronic illness, even people who have never considered this dimension of experience before instinctively reach for a personal meaning in events that have disrupted their lives. Meaning helps us to see in the dark. It strengthens the will to live in us.[4]

A number of studies have reported how conversion causes changes in one's belief system when there is trauma. In 1980, L. T. Dennis researched forty-six individuals' conversion experiences in L'Abri, Switzerland. Reflecting on Dennis's study, Antti Oksanen writes:

An external event or circumstances can have a primary impact upon the individual's meaning system. The event may be a death of a loved one, which jars the meaning system and throws it out of balance and raises questions of ultimate meaning. In that case the crisis of meaning may be resolved through conversion. During the conversion experience the person accepts a new or alternative meaning system which he/she judges more plausible and capable of restoring the ground of meaning in his/her life.[5]

C. Ullman, after researching the religious conversion of forty individuals (ten Jewish Orthodox, ten Roman Catholics, ten Hare Krishna, and ten Baha'i) and thirty non-converts (fifteen Jewish and fifteen Catholic), concludes that approximately 80 percent of converts experience emotional turmoil just prior to their conversion experience. She arrived at this conclusion after measuring levels of personal stress two years prior to conversion.[6] S. Syrjanen studied thirty-six individuals who converted from Islam to Christianity in Pakistan. After interviewing his subjects, he concluded that as many as 72 percent experienced various types of crises prior to or at the time of their conversion.[7]

Illness can cause similar results; it can provoke existential angst and questions about the meaning of being itself. Andre Samson, professor in the Department of Education at the University of Ottawa, and Chaplain Barbara Zerter capture the existential significance of the impact of illness when they write:

Illness can thus signify a threat to life, physical well-being, self-concept, social and occupational functioning, values, commitments, emotional equilibrium, and belief systems. A reminder of human vulnerability, it can provoke an existential crisis. Illness profoundly challenges a person's sense of purpose and meaning in life, raising fundamental questions of meaning, the nature of suffering and personal and social responses to it. It provokes the existential question of why this is happening to them. The spiritual challenge of illness . . . is to find a response to these questions.[8]

One of the findings of Samson and Zerter's study of cancer patients shows that their encounters with cancer led to an intense awareness of finiteness. With the experience of finiteness come questions of meaning, illness, and life itself. According to Samson and Zerter, the study confirms the centrality of human beings' quest for meaning. It demonstrates that "the subjects face two questions of meaning: the meaning or purpose of their illness, and the broader meaning of their life. Their quest begins with their efforts to find meaning for their illness."[9]

Elizabeth Johnston Taylor's qualitative study of spiritual needs among twenty-three patients with cancer and their family caregivers identified seven categories: the need to relate to the Ultimate Other for positivity and hope; for love (giving and receiving); to review beliefs; to create meaning; for religious rituals; and, finally, to prepare for death. Relating to the developmental task are her questions regarding the need to review beliefs and create meaning, such as: "ask 'why' questions," get over or get past asking 'why me,'" "find helpful explanations for why this illness happened," "become aware of positive things that have come with this illness," "sense that there is a reason for being alive now," "try to make life count," and "reevaluate your life."[10]

Reflecting on the coping strategies of rape victims, Kristen Leslie writes, "We live in trauma until we can reorganize, classify, and make sense of it."[11]

Transition

What takes place when an individual is confronted with severe illness or loss? As stated previously, the task is to integrate "nonbeing" (pain, suffering, and mortality) into one's system of meaning and beliefs. How does this take place? What does a person have to do? Individuals who cope well are those who make the transition from initial resistance to acceptance of their state of being. This transition often moves in the opposite direction of our society. We live in a fix-it society that does not leave much room for negativity and nonbeing. We prefer high self-esteem, perfect health, long life, and great romance. We crave "being" and shy away from the need to accommodate "nonbeing." We push negative thoughts away. We suppress. We hide. We admire the slim, fit, strong, smart, and smooth. We despise the ugly, the stupid, the clumsy, and the weak. Yet both extremes exist in all of us at some level. Our culture does not promote acceptance of these multiple dimensions of human vulnerability. But it seems to me that healthy people are those who learn to accept and integrate pain and suffering into their system of meaning, because ultimately there is no life without death, no health without sickness, and no pleasure without pain. The belief system of an individual who has gone through the lesson of pain is often more complex and sophisticated, with a higher threshold level for the harsh reality that life may present.

In many ways, life is a journey toward acceptance. Elizabeth Kubler-Ross, through her research with dying patients, helps us understand the stages they go through and the movement and transition from denial to acceptance.[12] These stages may be applicable to many other areas of life as well.

I once heard a story about a pastor who loved to conduct marriage and family seminars. After he got married, he stopped conducting them but he still loved conducting parenting seminars. After he and his wife had children, those seminars stopped as well. There was a missionary in my hometown who wanted to tell others how to raise children. He had two beautiful, obedient girls. Then he had a son who was not as obedient, and he no longer had any desire to educate others about raising children. I remember seeing a mother and son in a fast-food restaurant many years ago. The son said to his mom, "I want to eat chicken." And for some reason the mother did not want him to eat chicken. "No, you can't," she said. He spoke louder and she kept saying no. Then he started yelling. Out of anger, she turned to him and squeezed his mouth, shaking it vigorously. I remember sitting there and thinking to myself, "Yes, he is naughty, but how can a mother do that to her son?" Not long after, I had a son. Then I thought, "How can he do this to his mother?"

After counseling a number of couples, I learned that the journey they go through is a movement toward acceptance. Married life starts with expectations. With time, life teaches one to learn acceptance or to go insane. And often, in a strange way, in giving up expectations, conflicts are resolved and we come to realize that things do get better. Life is a journey, and illness initiates us into the process. It propels us from a simple to a complex understanding of self and the world. Life moves toward reality and greater complexity. According to my wife's profound philosophy, "The more complex our belief system, the more able we become at living a simple life." Chinese sages have said, "Life is trying to tell us something. Listen to life." But they add, "When a student is ready, a teacher will appear." And when we have learned from life—from listening to life carefully—we may finally discover what Henri Nouwen calls ecstasy:

It is a joy that does not separate happy days from sad days, successful moments from moments of failure, experiences of honor from experiences of dishonor, passion from resurrection. This joy is a divine gift that does not leave us during times of illness, poverty, oppression, or persecution. It is present even when the world laughs or tortures, robs or maims, fights or kills. It is truly ecstatic, always moving us away from the house of fear into the house of love, and always proclaiming that death no longer has the final say.[13]

Reflecting on their study of individuals with chronic illness, Marja Ohman, Siv Soderberg, and Berit Lundman write: "Once the individual has accepted what was endured, then suffering ceases and the person is in the process of acceptance and a reformulation of the self."[14]

This process influences theological views as well. For individuals struggling with a life-threatening diagnosis, over time there seems to be a shift from believing in an all-powerful God who intervenes through miracles to an understanding of God as the One who offers strength and comfort through times of trial, from the God who removes suffering to the God who remains through suffering. This change in theological perspective reflects the integration process and the embracing of negative elements into the system of meaning. It is in this restructuring of theology that sustenance of meaning in the face of finiteness, mortality, suffering, and death becomes possible.

Figure 3: Faith Journey

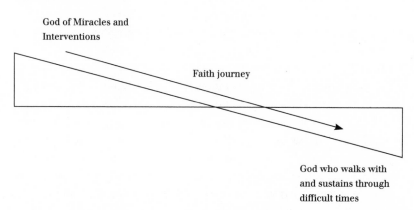

God of Miracles and
Interventions

Faith journey

God who walks with
and sustains through
difficult times

When my dad first learned that his cancer had metastasized, his theological stance was initially for God's intervention. He refused to believe otherwise. As time passed, he got worse and gradually came to see God as the One who offered strength and courage. However, he wanted very much to be a witness, to be cheerful and upbeat even in the face of death, and when sadness overwhelmed him, he felt disappointed with himself. He wanted to sing and laugh and be courageous, but he was, at the same time, sad and frightened and depressed. On his deathbed, as friends gathered, he said:

I thought I ought to be strong. I thought I ought to smile and be cheerful. I thought I ought to be an example of faith and not let this fear affect me. I tried. I tried really hard. But I did not succeed. When I try to smile, I feel my tears. When I try to project courage, I am overwhelmed with fear. When I try to laugh, I cannot convince myself of its humor. I am afraid. I am sad. I am confused, and I learned through this entire experience that it is all right. It is all right to be afraid, to feel sad, to worry and have faith in God at the same time.[15]

Just before he passed away, my dad came to fully integrate finiteness into his theological perspective. He learned that it is all right to be sad and to have faith at the same time. It is all right to be discouraged and to trust God at the same time, and to be depressed and to know that God will always remain by your side. This theological shift makes the integration of nonbeing into one's system of meaning possible.

Rabbi Kushner, the author of the best-selling *When Bad Things Happen to Good People*, was a believer in an all-powerful God who was in control of human destiny until he lost his fourteen-year-old son to an incurable disease.[16] Reflecting on the Twenty-third Psalm, Kushner writes, "The 23rd offers lessons on gratitude ('My cup runneth over'), direction ('he guides me in straight paths for his name's sake'), and inner peace ('he makes me to lie down in green pastures'). It doesn't say 'I will fear no evil' because evil only happens to bad people," Kushner says. "It says there is a lot of evil out there, but I can handle it because God is on my side."[17] The events of September 11, according to Kushner, have deepened his understanding of the meaning of this psalm. "God's promise is that whenever we have to confront the unfairness of life, he will be with us."[18]

Research

In support of this perspective, I will cite several social science studies.

Sociologist David Karp's qualitative study of fifty individuals with chronic depression concludes by documenting the four stages depressed people go through. In the first stage, depressed people think that something outside themselves has caused their depression. It can be their spouse, their living condition, their work situation, or their support system. Over time they come to realize that even when the external variables are dealt with or removed, depression remains. This awareness leads to the second stage. In stage two, depressed people come to recognize that they have depression and there is nothing they can blame for it. Stage two is often a short stage, and they move on to stage three, during which they start searching and experimenting with psychotropic medications and therapeutic modalities or looking for the best therapist to cure them of their melancholia. This, according to Karp, is often the longest stage. Often they come to the realization that their depression is chronic; that no matter what they do, they still have to live with depression at some level or with the possibility of another cycle of depression. This acceptance, according to Karp, is common among people who suffer chronic depression, and is probably the most spiritual stage. Depression often becomes more manageable with acceptance. The world takes on a different meaning. The person with chronic depression regains a sense of purpose.[19]

Johnny Ramirez Johnson, Carlos Fayard, Carlos Garberoglio, and Clara Jorge Ramirez's research on the relationship between faith and emotion among fifty-eight breast cancer patients reveals interesting findings. Emotion plays a significant role in how breast cancer patients define faith. Using six basic emotions (positive: love, joy, surprise; negative: anger, sadness, fear), this study finds that most patients report positive emotions (82.9%) in relation to their faith. However, it is interesting to note that negative emotions (fear and sadness) are also part of their faith expression. These negative emotions correlate with intrinsic religious motivation as well: "The fact that negative emotion words were used at all indicates the need to understand religious faith as a construct that encompasses negative as well as positive emotions."[20]

Jenenne Nelson's phenomenological study of the experience of uncertainty among nine breast cancer patients (ages 38–69) two to six years post-treatment shows a number of interesting findings. The sense of uncertainty they experienced presented itself as a challenge for them to try to find new ways of being in the world. In dealing with uncertainty itself, they have to come to terms with trying to understand their disease in a broader and more meaningful perspective.[21]

Bryn Seyle's and my qualitative study of theological strategies, meaning, and coping among participants with breast cancer reveals similar findings. Individuals who believe in miraculous intervention and wait for miracles to happen recover more slowly and do not seem to cope as well as individuals who accept cancer as a part of reality and who believe cancer can happen to anyone. A breast cancer patient reflects:

I don't think it was an act of God . . . nor was it anything personal. And when I look back I don't think there was anything I could have done otherwise to have prevented it. . . . What else I could have done differently, I don't know. It could have been genetic . . . it was just one of those things. . . . To me, cancer doesn't discriminate between race, sex, religion . . . the young, the poor. . . . It happened and I accepted it, and I guess I just want to move on more than anything else. I just don't want to waste too much time and energy trying to figure it out. . . . It's like one of those profound things in life like "why am I here, what is the purpose of my life?"[22]

There also seems to be an indication that people who come to terms with cancer often had prior experiences with major loss or trauma that in some way prepared them to cope with new trauma. A physician who was diagnosed with breast cancer states:

I think prior to my diagnosis of cancer I knew that bad things happen to good people, and I had experiences in my childhood with losing my father, losing my brother at a young age and seeing other family members go through very difficult things. . . . Prior to my diagnosis of cancer I watched my mother-in-law, who I think is just one of the most wonderful saintly Christian woman in the world, go through a horrible experience with cancer, and I guess I had to reconcile some of those issues of why bad things happened at that point . . . and again I came to the point of feeling that this was not something that God wanted, this was not something that God caused, but there is evil in the world, and that this is a consequence of evil in the world.

While the first group finds meaning in making the connection between God and the illness (God is the cause of cancer for a reason), the second group does not posit God as the cause, believing that cancer can happen to anyone. Women in this group believe that God has a plan but often admit that they are not aware of God's plan for their lives. The final group's belief system, however, is not affected by cancer. Their lives are meaningful with or without cancer. They seem to be able to locate meaning in the midst of pain and suffering itself and therefore do not need an explanation for what they are going through.[23]

A qualitative study on the relationship between chronic pain and meaning among fifteen chronic pain patients by Kelvin Thompson, Leigh Aveling, Art Earll, and me, shows that prior to admission to the pain track program at Loma Linda University Behavioral Medicine Center, most participants defined meaning as the ability to engage in productive activities and positive relationship. In other words, they defined meaning as a lack of negative elements. With the onset of chronic pain, they experienced multiple losses in many areas of their lives, such as outdoor activities, relationships, and careers. Often their initial attempt to regain a sense of meaning was through medication. Prescription drugs initially helped to alleviate their pain and enabled them to resume their prior meaningful activities, thus helping them retain a sense of meaning. However, over time they become dependent on and even addicted to their medications. Addiction only makes things worse and creates many other sets of problems. For these participants recovery comes when they acquire a more complex understanding of themselves that explains the relationship between emotion, pain, and addiction. This includes their ability to see the connection between pain and unresolved emotion and guilt, and the realization that they cannot force life to move in the direction of their definition of meaning. These individuals do not define a meaningful life and pursue that definition; they see life as it comes and create meaning within their present situations. They have come to realize that pain and meaning can coexist. As one participant commented, "I mean it's always going to be there. It's something that is not going away." Spirituality enhances one's ability to let go and live in the present, even in the midst of pain. A female participant who had been living with pain for over ten years finally came to recognize, "It's learning to live life on life's terms."[24]

While interviewing ten women infected with AIDS in northern Thailand, I noticed the strength that religion brought to the lives of some of these individuals. Of the ten, six reported suicidal ideation. But the four who did not experience suicidal thoughts indicated a firm belief in the Buddhist concept of karma, that the length of one's life depends on merits one acquired in the previous life. According to this Buddhist teaching, acceptance of the finality of life was firmly rooted in the psyche of these four participants. One informant reflected, "Every one of us has to die at some point. For some it is sooner and for others, later. No one can escape death. I just happen to be the unlucky one."[25]

Conclusion

Often individuals who are confronted with trauma initially seek to eliminate suffering because they are not able to see how the senselessness of suffering can be meaningful and how they can continue to live a meaningful life. However, through time, the task they have to deal with is to learn to integrate suffering and mortality into their system of meaning or face the alternative of moving on in life with no possibility of regaining meaning. This is where spirituality plays a significant role. When our current system is no longer able to sustain us, spirituality will urge us to move forward, to reconfigure our understanding of reality and God in order to regain meaning and purpose. Pain is bearable, but lack of meaning is unimaginable. Through this profound invitation of the spirit, often individuals will come to the place of acceptance of their situation in life. It is in acceptance that healing takes place. Albert Y. Hsu, reflecting on the tragic death of his father, concludes, "Despite all our questioning, perhaps there simply aren't any answers to the why questions. Maybe we don't know why and we can't know why. Maybe that's all we know."[26] Perhaps it is best to conclude with words from a person who understands, existentially, the meaning of cancer. Columnist Jory Graham writes:

The way to find meaning in an absurd situation is to take some kind of action. My action was a search for a different perspective on *why me?* because the question is so loaded with implications of injustice. Since I could not blame God, or myself, or the polluters of our environment, I was confounded—and angry. I didn't know why I had cancer (I still don't), but the unfairness of losing my freedom and my life to it filled me with rage. . . .

Why not me? Who am I to be so special that I cannot get cancer? Who am I to be so egocentric as to believe that random luck is for others, but not for me? From then on, it is only a matter of time to *it is me*, and, *what am I going to do now?* With this question comes a feeling of enlightenment and a sense of power.[27]

CHAPTER FIVE

Integration in Theology and Religious Symbols

Pleasure and rage

Sadness and joy

Hopes and regrets

Change and stability

Weakness and decision

Impatience and sloth:

All are sounds from the same flute,

All mushrooms from the same wet mould.

—Chuang Tzu

The previous chapter discusses the developmental task patients often need to undertake, a process of integration that leads them to find a sense of meaning in suffering itself. Social science research examples supported the developmental task concept. This chapter discusses the same concept from the standpoint of our rich theological and religious literary traditions, which also affirm integration as essential. Our discussion will include summaries and excerpts from the writings of Paul Tillich, John Macquarrie, Dietrich Bonhoeffer, and, finally, a detailed outline based on the work of Raimundo Panikkar. The section that examines religious symbolism as a representation of integration will include a discussion of yin and yang within the Taoist worldview, alchemy (as explained by Carl Jung), and an Indian goddess.

Integration in Theological Literature

Facing life-threatening or chronic illness often raises theological issues in the minds of those who are in the midst of this existential struggle. As stated in the previous chapter, it is not uncommon for people with breast cancer or chronic pain to ask theological questions and ultimately experience theological (or worldview) transformation, mirroring contemporary theological and religious perspectives. Perhaps theology and religion are attempts to reconfigure concepts in ways that speak to the present reality of the world we live in and, for this very reason, religious symbolism speaks of the need to integrate negative elements into belief systems.

Paul Tillich

As stated in chapter one, Tillich sees the person of Christ as the place of integration. Belief in Christ enables one to accept and face the negative aspects in life because, to Tillich, Christ as the final revelation of God refused to give in to the threat of nonbeing. He refused to allow the fear of death itself to distract him from his mission. Christ insisted on love even when death was inevitable. He accepted its reality and embraced it. He faced it with courage and, by so doing, authenticated life itself without giving in to despair. Human beings in a state of existential estrangement cannot restore themselves and regain their essential state of being. The only way is through revelation, which takes place in the New Being. This New Being is symbolized in the person of Christ. Christ reflects the New Being because, although he took on all the infirmities of human finitude, he conquered them through courage in the face of nonbeing.[1] "Although he has only finite freedom," writes Tillich, "he is not estranged from the ground of his being."[2] Through Christ as the symbol of New Being, human beings can now accept their finitude and the negativities inherent within it without rebellion. In *The Courage to Be*, Tillich writes:

Courage is the self-affirmation of being in spite of the fact of nonbeing. It is the act of the individual self in taking the anxiety of nonbeing upon itself by affirming itself either as part of an embracing whole or in its individual selfhood. Courage always includes a risk, it is always threatened by nonbeing, whether the risk of losing oneself and becoming a thing within the whole of things or of losing one's world in an empty self-relatedness. Courage needs the power of being, a power transcending the nonbeing which is experienced in the anxiety of fate and death, which is present in the anxiety of emptiness and meaninglessness, which is effective in the anxiety of guilt and condemnation.[3]

John Macquarrie

We see a similar approach in the writings of John Macquarrie, who, in his *Principles of Christian Theology*, suggests that God is Being. In the process of creation, God gives God's life into nothingness. Human beings and the world of creation are finite beings given by God. This "giving of self" into nothingness takes the form of evolution. "Again, the process of evolution on the earth's surface looks more like a groping procedure of trial and error, with fantastic waste."[4] Human beings as given by God in God's act of self-giving must struggle through this evolutionary process in their quest for true self-hood. An individual in his/her "freedom and responsibility, has a share of creativity and cooperates with God in the shaping of the world."[5] Human beings need to face their finiteness, embrace it fully, and work within its limits to bring about a better world through the blessing of God. Macquarrie calls this struggle for affirmation love, the love of "Jesus Christ as absolute letting-be."[6] Macquarrie offers a passionate perspective on theology that fully embraces human finiteness.

Dietrich Bonhoeffer

In *Letters and Papers from Prison*, Dietrich Bonhoeffer argues that the God of the gap, the God whose power starts at the edge of human limitations, is merely a projection of human fantasy. This God only perpetuates human inclinations and does not in any way challenge a person to grow and be responsible. He states that the weak God is the only God who can save. Bonhoeffer believes that as Christians we should learn to live totally in this world, accept what comes with it, and learn to live responsibly.

God would have us know that we must live as men who manage our lives without him. The God who is with us is the God who forsakes us (Mark 15:34). The God who lets us live in the world without the working hypothesis of God is the

God before whom we stand continually. Before God and with God we live without God. God lets himself be pushed out of the world on to the cross. He is weak
and powerless in the world, and that is precisely the way, the only way, in which
he is with us and helps us.[7]

For a more extensive conceptualization of this concept, I will turn
to an Asian theologian and philosopher, Raimundo Panikkar. Examining the concept in greater depth may help us recognize the significant
implications of this approach in theology.

Raimundo Panikkar

Panikkar's integration of finiteness starts with his understanding of
God and the place of reason. To Panikkar, reason cannot construct an
understanding of reality that will provide meaning within the face of
nonbeing. The question is, how can one deal with this threat of nonbeing, mortality, and suffering? The answer regarding Ultimate Reality,
argues Panikkar, is not found in human rationality but rather is implied
in the silence and smile of the Buddha.

God

God cannot be known. The god that can be known is not God. This
echoes Lao Tzu's teaching that the way that can be "wayed" is not
the eternal way. God is God because God is beyond. God is beyond
the realm of logos and concepts: "I Am that I Am." The recognition of
this leads one to a better understanding of the silence of the Buddha
regarding ultimate truth or God. When asked about the Absolute, Buddha kept silence. His silence did not make him an agnostic, but identified him as an enlightened one. What is the implication of the Buddha's
silence?

Silence implies that the answer regarding the Absolute does not exist
because we are relative, limited, and contingent. Any attempt to name
God will only be a projection. Buddha wants us to come to know and
appreciate this silence. Silence invites us to move beyond the world's
signs, words, speech, and logos. "Without myth, the *logos* becomes absolute, it divinizes itself, and a divinized *logos* destroys itself."[8]

Silence was not the Buddha's answer. He aimed to silence the question itself. We are to silence the question because it has no meaning.

"What the Buddha requires is a realistic sense of acceptance of reality just as it presents itself, a total confidence in life, in what is given to us, without seeking to replace Reality with our own ideas."[9] We are invited to "total acceptance of our human condition, of the real contingency in which we find ourselves," because to "thirst is to transgress Reality, to evade the human situation."[10] The real contingency of ourselves needs to be embraced. This is not about resignation but connotes accepting and bettering it. In letting go of this thirst, human beings can regain innocence once more. In silencing the question, Panikkar begs us to silence the logos as well, because God belongs to the realm that transcends our categories of thinking. Panikkar concludes that in helping us come to appreciate silence, "The Buddha smiles!"[11]

Truth and Liberation

If the Absolute, which belongs to the realm that transcends our categories of thinking and contingency, is the fact of life we have to face: What is the meaning of truth? How can we even think of verifying truth? What is truth? Truth is something that is true in itself. It is infallibility. "The rational affirmation of infallibility leads to solipsism. . . . This amounts to saying that infallibility is unverifiable, that infallibility has no other basis than its own self-affirmation. . . . Infallibility belongs to the order of myth."[12] Myth is not an object but an instrument of knowing and an attitude. When we make myth an object of knowledge, we destroy myth. This concept of myth reflects an "inner connection" within the structure of being that transcends logic. It is intuitive in nature. Reality cannot be limited to what can be grasped only by our reasoning. Myth connects us to the reality within ourselves and the world around us. "Myth gives us a reference point that orients us in reality." Seeing myth as something that connects us with our inner reality suggests the universal quest within humanity for the authenticity of the self. Myth is universal, and its universality reflects an element within the structure of human beings seeking to direct the self toward the quintessence of being itself.[13] That's why Panikkar writes, "Humankind cannot live without myth."[14]

This definition implies that if truth, which is infallible, seeks verification outside of itself, it becomes fallible. "To say 'this act is infallible' amounts to saying 'this act has in itself its own principle of verification.'"[15]

If this is so, how can infallibility verify itself? Panikkar's answer is that it has to emerge from the very same ground. The quest for religious truth and meaning emerges from humanity and, therefore, humanity itself becomes this very ground of verification. In speaking of infallibility, Panikkar makes the distinction between epistemological and ontological infallibility. In epistemological infallibility, there is no point outside or above it. Thus, it becomes a truism, because there is nothing outside of humanity that can be the judge. Ontological infallibility acknowledges a transcendent reference point. This model becomes the "expression of a hope, since it is quite conceivable that humanity could 'fall', 'fail' and not accomplish its destiny, not fulfill itself."[16] How can humanity verify its infallibility? What constitutes religion, suggests Panikkar, is not doctrines but actions. As such, infallibility is grounded in praxis. Infallibility is not a theory, but the life one lives. It is having confidence in life and believing in the meaning of human existence. In describing *orthopraxis* (right practice), Panikkar writes: "Authentic infallibility entails the most complete assumption of risk, for the greatest risk is to accept the infallibility of each moment of our life, fully aware that the next moment may well bring another insight because a new reality dawns upon us and not because . . . we refrain from exhausting the present."[17]

We need to dare to believe strongly in the meaning of our existence and act on it. This very act will save us. It is this praxis that makes us infallible. And this is the essence of religious truth. Religion is salvific. Religion claims to liberate. Salvation and liberation take place through action. "Man must employ, discover, believe, initiate, put into practice, etc., in order to attain his salvation, destiny, end, goal."[18] To be saved is to be free. To be free is to be liberated. To be liberated means to be "liberated from" and "liberated to." In other words, we need to be "free from" and "free to" in order to claim freedom. To be free implies freedom from all limitations, to be free from the sufferings, fears, doubts, anxieties, and insecurities of life. To be free from all limitations also implies freedom from religion itself. When religion binds a person through fear and obligation, that person is not truly free. To be free, therefore, is to be existentially free. This existential freedom takes place when one is free also from religion and free from God. In fact, God wants us to be free from God so that we may be free for God. Christ is this very symbol of freedom. According to Panikkar, "Christ is the principle of freedom illumining every Man coming into this world; he came to tell us we must judge for ourselves, shoulder our responsibilities, bring our given talents to fruition, and learn to forgive . . . by our participation in the creative act of forgiving, we give life to ourselves and to others."[19]

Religious truth, therefore, is to be found in humanity affirming itself through praxis based on freedom. Panikkar writes, "The act of ontically exercising freedom is the religious act by which man is saved (or doomed). The religious act is the act of freedom."[20]

Reflecting on Panikkar's understanding of religion leads me to believe that the desired freedom is freedom from the conditions of life that inauthenticate life itself. Only through freedom can being truly be. Only through freedom can authenticity become a possibility. The achievement of this freedom is reflected in the teachings of Jesus when he said, "For whoever wants to save his life will lose it, but whoever loses his life for me and for the gospel will save it" (Mark 8:35). Hsiang-Kuo, a Neo-Taoist, expresses a similar concept: "The Tao is everywhere, but everywhere it is nothing."[21] Also in his commentary on the Chuang-tzu, he states:

In existence, what is prior to things? We say that Yin and Yang are prior to things. But the Yin and Yang are themselves things; what then, is prior to the Yin and Yang? We may say that Tzu Jan [nature or naturalness] is prior to things. But Tzu Jan is simply the naturalness of things. Or we may say that the Tao is prior to things. But the Tao is nothing. Since it is nothing, how can it be prior to things? We do not know what is prior to things, yet things are continuously produced. This shows that things are spontaneously what they are; there is no Creator of things.[22]

The basis of human freedom is the finiteness of being where time is temporal and space is limited. Pain and suffering remind us of our nonbeing and finiteness. We are like grass in the field. The acceptance of nonbeing is "encountering Being." To face the finiteness of our being is to come face-to-face with God. To face nonbeing, in essence, is an invitation to spirituality. In the face of death, one awakens to the deeper meaning of life. To Panikkar, only through our willingness to give our lives are we able to regain the authenticity of the self. Panikkar confirms the most powerful symbol of Christianity when he suggests that true spirituality, the achievement of the "freedom to be," takes place when one is willing to lay down one's life. True spirituality is contained in the symbol of the cross.

Summary

In summary, we can say that spirituality is rooted in the fact that we are finite and yet within this finiteness there is something transcendental within our ontological structure. This finiteness would not have provoked a spiritual quest but human beings have the ability to self-define through self-awareness. The awareness of finiteness and infinity within being, in the face of the possibility of nonbeing, provokes the anxiety of the soul. In despair, we often strive to grasp the Absolute as a source of security, not realizing that what we grasp is just a fragment projected from the contingency of our lives. And we start dictating to this "grasped absolute" by placing God in the categories of space, time, and human logos. In this process, we inauthenticate life. The task of spirituality is not to grasp the Absolute but to appreciate the silence and remain in mystery. The question no longer exists, but God remains. Or, as Ann Ulanov puts it, "We need a consciousness that can tolerate not-knowing."[23] The task of spirituality is to find meaning within the face of nonbeing. Where is the source of healing? Religious truth is believed to be the source because religions provide salvation. To be saved is to be free. Freedom implies that, at the cross, destiny has been given into the hands of humanity. Essence does not precede existence. Here, human engagement in praxis is the only ground for the verification of truth. Truth is verified when we intentionally engage ourselves in changing human reality. The act of exercising freedom is the religious act whereby we will either be saved or lost. The call to spirituality is a call to the task of finding meaning in the face of nonbeing on the basis of freedom (or liberation/salvation) obtained through "religion." Therefore, according to Panikkar, religious truth liberates us from the anxiety of being through embracing nonbeing, accepting mystery, and exercising freedom through engaging in the reality of life.

Religious Symbols

When life seems senseless, people turn to religion because religion has the potential to offer meaning even in the face of death itself. For this reason, wisdom from world religions seems to point as well to the integration of being and nonbeing, the need to assimilate vulnerabilities and human finiteness into an affirmation of meaning in humanity. In *Bhagavad Gita,* Krishna offers this advice: "Be in truth eternal, beyond earthly opposites!"[24] In describing the Eastern way of life, Fritjof Capra writes:

The notion that all opposites are polar—that light and dark, winning and losing, good and evil, are merely different aspects of the same phenomenon—is one of the basic principles of the Eastern way of life. Since all opposites are interdependent, their conflict can never result in the total victory of one side, but will always be a manifestation of the interplay between the two sides. In the East, a virtuous person is therefore not one who undertakes the impossible task of striving for the good and eliminating the bad, but rather one who is able to maintain a dynamic balance between good and bad.[25]

There are many ancient religious symbols that speak to this movement toward integration, including the mandala, the labyrinth, the *Kundalini* of Tantric Buddhism, the union of *lingum* and *yoni* in Hinduism, the nothingness or void that unites opposites in Taoism, to name a few. I will describe just three religious symbols of integration: yin and yang, Kali, and alchemy.

Yin and Yang

In Taoist philosophy, yin and yang symbolize the message of integration. There is light and darkness, good and bad, strength and weakness, laughter and sorrow, health and sickness, life and death. Lao Tzu teaches:

> Being and nonbeing produce each other;
> Difficult and easy complete each other;
> Long and short contrast each other;
> High and low distinguish each other;

> Sound and voice harmonize with each other;
> Front and back follow each other.[26]

All is a part of the one reality called the Tao. The Tao includes everything and excludes nothing. Wing-Tsit Chan describes the Tao thus: "It is at once the beginning of all things and the way in which all things pursue their course."[27] The problems we face in our lives are primarily because we are not willing to accept that life is both yin and yang, good and bad, health and sickness, joy and sadness. We want to control and manipulate. We want to eliminate all the negatives and, by doing so, we move away from the Way itself. We move away from ourselves and, as a result, become more and more inauthentic. For this reason, Taoism is an invitation to return to what is "the way it is."[28] Or, in the words of Nietzsche, "What returns, what finally comes home to me, is my own self."[29]

Goddess Kali

At first glance, this religious symbol may not appear to be a symbol of integration. Goddess Kali is represented in black with four arms. In one hand, she holds a sword, in another, the head of the demon she has slain. She wears earrings made of skulls and her body is smeared with blood. This image does not seem to represent anything but violence and vengeance. But to believers, this symbolism embraces a much deeper meaning about integration in the reality of life.

The image of Kali, in a variety of ways, teaches man that pain, sorrow, decay, death, and destruction are not to be overcome or conquered by denying them or explaining them away. Pain and sorrow are woven into the texture of man's life so thoroughly that to deny them is ultimately futile. For man to realize the fullness of his being, for man to exploit his potential as a human being, he must finally accept this dimension of existence. Kali's boon is freedom, the freedom of the child to revel in the moment, and it is won only after confrontation or acceptance of death. To ignore death, to pretend that one is physically immortal, to pretend that one's ego is the center of things, is to provoke Kali's mocking laughter. . . . To accept one's mortality is to be able to let go, to be able to sing, dance, and shout. Kali is Mother to her devotees not because she protects them from the way things really are but because she reveals to them their mortality and thus releases them to act fully and freely, releases them from the incredible, binding web of "adult" pretense, practicality, and rationality.[30]

Jung and Alchemy

In many ways, the difficulties in life force us to learn to modify, adjust, or accept to better cope with life. This, to Jung, is the process of alchemy. I remember a single mother raising a teenage son who said to me, "In the end, the only thing you can do is to love them and be there for them. There is nothing much more we can really do because they are going to be what they are going to be." As our conversation continued, she informed me that she used to try, for very good reasons, to teach her son to be what she thought was good for him. The harder she tried, the worse it became. "It was too painful," she recalled. Then, she concluded, "I finally had to learn to let go and trust God."

Alchemy as a struggle to integrate opposites, particularly in the image of the *coniunctio* (Latin for "union"), reflects life's journey. The study of Jung's approach to alchemy can enhance our understanding of the process of integration at the symbolic and psychological level. The popular understanding of alchemists is that they were misguided visionaries who longed to turn lead into gold. In his study of the psyche's attempts to integrate opposites, Carl Jung paid close attention to the concept of alchemy. His study led him to a different understanding. The pursuit of substance transformation was only one part of a much more sophisticated philosophical-psychological system of thought that included personal transformation, the external projection of psychic processes seeking spiritual transformation.[31]

One of the final stages in alchemical procedures was the *coniunctio oppositorum*, the union of opposites, in which separated materials with opposite qualities were united at last to create a wholly new, transformed substance.

The chemical *coniunctio* was symbolized again and again by images of sexual union and by the half-man, half-woman figure of the hermaphrodite. This shocking symbolism of a chemical operation made clear to Jung that the alchemist's *coniunctio* must point to something more, to a mystery that might never be fully known.

What does the *coniunctio* point to? It points to an inward union of male and female elements necessary for psychological and spiritual wholeness that leads to a capacity for true intimacy and relationship. It is the symbol of psychic wholeness. Although the symbol represents male/female union, this should not be taken literally but figuratively. Male and female represent the archetypal opposites in general, such as active/passive, conscious/unconscious, light/darkness, and destructive/constructive. *Coniunctio*, however sexual its symbolism, represents the union of any opposite qualities whose reconciliation leads to greater oneness within oneself and others. It is of great importance to the process of individuation. "According to Jung, alchemical stages are symbolic expressions of the stages of individuation; individuation being that process by which we move toward the integration of opposites, their transcendence and finally the bringing into consciousness of the Self."[32]

Conclusion

Support for the need to integrate nonbeing into one's existential understanding of reality is not only provided by social science research showing how individuals learn to come to see meaning within pain, suffering, and mortality itself. Life has a way of teaching us. Individuals who struggle with existential meaning within the reality of this world of laughter and sorrow, comfort and pain, life and death, arrive at a deeper and more complex understanding of life through the spiritual drive within the ontological structure. They come to see and recognize the need to embrace nonbeing within their own belief system, a need which finds its symbolism in alchemy, Christian existentialism, Kali, and Panikkar's praxis.

CHAPTER SIX

Spirituality and Integration in Mental Health

And Something's odd—within—
That person that I was—
And this One—do not feel the same—
Could it be Madness—this?

—Emily Dickinson

This chapter looks at the meaning of spirituality among those who suffer emotional and psychological pain and defines the place of spirituality as a process of finding meaning within the chaos of one's mental state. A consideration of cultural factors is brought into the configuration by offering a model of understanding that moves beyond the immediate social context. We will examine Jung's approach to the integration of shadow into one's understanding of self as an example of the process of integration, and conclude by defining mental health not as a state free from pain, but rather as a state of self that has come to terms with itself.

Madness and the Quest for Self

If spirituality is the ontological drive to make sense of who we are, the question emerging from the place of mental distress is: who are we as we descend into the abyss of madness? This devastating senselessness becomes a quest that engages our spirituality in the very depth of our being. When life wants to terminate itself and thoughts race, when the world is painted gray and guilt haunts us at every step, when death is an option and life is a dread, when the world seems odd and the mind is in chaos, we ask the same question over and over. Why? Why do I feel so wrong, so alienated, so alone, so trapped in the senselessness of my wandering mind? Why? How can I make sense of these strange emotions and thoughts? The intense need to make sense out of the senselessness of the intrapsychic process haunts and alienates us.

We gain insights into this intrapsychic drive to find meaning in mental illness through the life and work of Anton T. Boisen, who played a significant role in providing clinical training for ministers during the early years of the clinical pastoral education movement. His struggle with anxiety, inner conflicts, and a sense of failure contributed to his first psychotic breakdown and hospitalization in October 1920, for fifteen months. This was the first of subsequent psychotic episodes that he endured. Two years after the first episode he recounted, "At one time I succeeded in climbing into the sun, but through some clumsiness, managed to destroy the balance of things and my friends and relatives in the sun suffered heavily in consequence. Thousands and thousands of them lost their lives."[1] Having ideas of going to the sun and moon and experiencing death, rebirth, and reincarnation, Boisen suggests, may not merely reflect psychotic and hallucinatory features of mental illness. Observing these symptoms, he writes:

Ideas of self-sacrifice, of death, of world disaster, of mystical identification, of rebirth, of reincarnation, of prophetic mission are to be found not only in my case but in other acutely disturbed schizophrenics also. . . . Such ideas do have meaning. . . . The idea of self-sacrifice and death, which is most frequent in schizophrenic thinking, represents quite accurately the loss or renunciation of something of supreme value, with which schizophrenic disturbances commonly begin. The idea of world disaster is the magnification of the personal death experience until it assumes cosmic proportions. The idea of rebirth stands for the inner meaning of acute schizophrenia, that of attempted renewal, or reorganization. The prophetic urge represents the world-wide outreach of vital religion, while cosmic identification comes with the sudden opening of the eyes to a staggering new insight, that even the most commonplace person is a social being, important beyond his wildest dreams.[2]

Boisen's observation of common themes among schizophrenic patients reflects the intrapsychic need for meaning in the depth of mental illness. This is perhaps one of the main reasons why religion plays a significant role in the way this population copes with pain. I recall a moment of profound insight while conversing with Kathleen Greider, professor of pastoral care and counseling at Claremont School of Theology. After she presented her research on spirituality among mentally ill patients to a group of medical students at Loma Linda University, I asked her to explain further the reason why this population turns to metaphors as a way of dealing with their pain. From our conversation I learned that everyday language is unable to accommodate their illness; it does not provide ways to articulate the emotional anguish and pain they go through.

Everyday language is confined within the boundary of logic. People do not walk through closed doors, fly in the sky, defy death, or predict the future. Experiences of mental illness move beyond logic. But metaphors make articulation possible. Metaphors move beyond logic and therefore create the possibility of meaning within chaos. This explains the role of religious symbols. Religion speaks of the world beyond and the world that transcends logic and reasoning. Religion enters the realm of metaphysics. In everyday language, mentally ill patients are simply crazy and mad in the most senseless way. In religion, there is a possibility that something exists beyond this world, beyond the physical—a world where they are more than just mad. In religion, there is a possibility that their experiences may be meaningful. The life of Sri Bhagavan Maharshi (1879–1950), an important Tamil saint, is one such example. At the age of sixteen, he was overcome with a fear of death. This experience drove him to seek answers to the meaning of death itself, and he finally discovered that death only touches the body, not the soul. After this experience, he no longer had any interest in school, friends, or any regular activities. He left his family and moved from temple to temple, living a life of almost complete silence and immobility and neglecting his body to the extreme. Describing the Bhagavan's situation in the temple, A. Osborne writes:

The floor of the shrine was infected with ants but he seemed oblivious to their crawling over him and biting him. After some time a stool was placed in the corner for him to sit on and its legs immersed in water to keep them away, but even then he leaned back against the wall and so made a bridge for them. From constant sitting there his back made a permanent imprint on the wall. . . . [His] body was utterly neglected. He ignored it completely. It was unwashed; his hair had grown again and was thick and matted; his finger nails had grown long and curled over. . . . His body was weakened to the limit of endurance. When he needed to go out he had barely the strength to rise. He would raise himself up a few inches and then sink back again, weak and dizzy, and would have to try several times before he could rise to his feet.[3]

The Bhagavan's life, particularly his two years of complete withdrawal, may be viewed as a psychotic episode. But he became known as a great spiritual leader, a saint, well respected in India and around the world as well.[4] A saint or a madman? While everyday language and social norms (in Western society, in particular) can only view this behavior as deviation, religion offers meaning. Religion can potentially provide sense to senselessness and meaning to madness.

Similarly, we see expressions of deep emotion beyond the realm of the ordinary through art, music, and poetry. Somewhere in the deeper self lie irrational feelings, real and frightening and far from the spoken words of everyday language. Yet this madness is capable of generating much profoundness in the quest for spirituality. In the words of Henry James Sr., "The natural inheritance of everyone who is capable of spiritual life is an unsubdued forest where the wolf howls and the obscene bird of night chatters."[5]

In her book *Undercurrents*, Martha Manning recounts her struggle with depression:

I pray the prayers long quiet on my tongue, but so easily retrieved. The recitation is a continual battle between despair and hope, death and life. The thoughts of guns and ropes and pills keep coming. I close my eyes to them, trying to squeeze them out of awareness.

> Hail Mary, full of grace . . .
> Block out of the thoughts, Martha. Shut out the pain.
> The Lord is with thee . . .
> I can't do this. I can't go on.
> Blessed art thou among women . . .
> Please, just let me die.
> And blessed is the fruit of thy womb, Jesus.
> Jesus, where are you?

Keep going. Through the Hail Marys and the Our Fathers and the Glory Be's. Just say the words. Just keep saying them. Over and over and over again. Till the prayers find their way to heaven and I am blessed, finally, with the mercy of sleep.[6]

The movement toward metaphor, art, poetry, and religion is a movement toward the possibility of meaning in chaos, purpose in madness; a suffocated self struggling for air.

Defining Mental Health: The Problem

We need to discuss a couple of important issues as we explore the place of integration in the lives of those who struggle with emotional pain. First, there is the task of defining mental health. What is mental health? Is it possible to be mad in one culture and sane in the other, to be rude in one and gentle in the other, to be antisocial in one and spiritual in another? What is sanity? What is madness? Gerald May writes, "In the midst of every dimension of delusion there are sparkles of sanity."[7]

Cultural variance in the experience of mental illness is well documented. Among the Plains Indians, hearing voices from loved ones who have just passed away is a common experience and is therefore non-pathological within the practice of the community. However, an adult, white North American having a similar experience is considered delusional and viewed as suffering from serious mental anguish.[8] Studies of schizophrenia seem to suggest a certain level of universality due to a similarity in symptoms across cultures, such as hallucinations, delusions, withdrawal, and impaired reality testing. However, epidemiological and ethnographic studies show that this illness is not equally distributed. "The prevalence ranges from 1 in 1,000 in non-Western societies to more than 1 in 100 in Western societies."[9] There is a higher rate of schizophrenia in economically advanced urban societies than in peasant societies. Furthermore, schizophrenia in India tends to be catatonic but it is not in Western Europe and America. In China and Nigeria, the onset of schizophrenia is more rapid than in the United States. Studies by the World Health Organization suggest that schizophrenia in poor countries is often not as serious and shows better outcomes.[10] Among the Zulus, the shaman is the person who is delicate, constantly complains of pain, experiences convulsions, gets teary, and cries noisily when not respected.[11]

One of the most extensive cross-cultural studies on depression by the World Health Organization based on 573 patients from five countries (Canada, India, Iran, Japan, and Switzerland) supports the importance of social context on mental health. Guilt feelings are present in 68 percent of the Swiss sample, but only 32 percent in the Iranian sample. Seventy percent of Canadian subjects experience suicidal ideation, but only 40 percent do among the Japanese sample. Fifty-seven percent of the Iranian sample reported somatization, which is present among only 27 percent of the Canadian sample.[12] "Reviewers concur that feelings of guilt, self-deprecation, suicidal ideas, and feelings of despair are often rare or absent among non-European populations, whereas somatic and quasi-somatic symptoms, including disturbances of sleep, appetite, energy, body sensation, and motor function, are more common."[13]

Reflecting on these cross-cultural studies on psychiatric illness, Arthur Kleinman states:

Of all the adult mental disorders described in DSM-IV, besides the organic brain disorders and substance abuse, convincing evidence supports the case of only four that are distributed worldwide: schizophrenia, manic-depressive (bipolar) disorder, major depression, and a group of anxiety disorders including panic anxiety, obsessive-compulsive disorder, and certain phobias. The rest of our adult mental illness categories are peculiar to North America and Western Europe. An interesting example is anorexia nervosa. This disorder exists in contemporary Western societies that regard slim female bodies as beautiful, sexually desirable, and commercially significant. Except among the Westernized upper middle class of Japan, Taiwan, and Hong Kong, there is no anorexia nervosa in Asia.[14]

Besides cultural issues, there are sociological and political issues involved in the way we understand psychology as well. Exploring the political and social agenda in psychopathology, Rachel Hare-Mustin and Jeanne Marecek write:

The relation of psychiatric diagnoses to culture, societal structure, and historical circumstance is readily apparent if we look at times and places other than our own. Before the emancipation of slaves in the United States, for example, the term "drapetomania" was promoted as a diagnostic label for slaves' uncontrollable urge to escape from slavery. Another example is the diagnosis of kleptomania, which refers to an irresistible compulsion to shoplift or pilfer. The diagnostic term "kleptomania" originated concurrently with the emergence of large department stores in European cities at the turn of the century. These stores afforded shoppers—who were mainly women—anonymity, an array of tempting merchandise, and the freedom to touch and handle items for sale. This created not only incentives to purchase, but also temptations to steal. Shoppers of all social classes stole, but authorities used social class to distinguish criminal acts of theft from those purportedly reflecting mental pathology. To put it bluntly, ordinary women were regarded as thieves, but upper-class women's acts of theft were explained as a product of mental illness.[15]

Perhaps we need to be aware of the role our assumptions play in the way we see others and define madness, in the way we draw bell curves and call others abnormal, and in the way we set norms and calculate standard deviations. That is to say, who is in and who is out, who is right and who is wrong? Who is normal and who is not? If we recognize the possibility of defining something normative as beyond the acceptable, we admit the limits of our assumptions. This recognition moves us to a higher level of self-awareness and a more encompassing transcultural definition of mental health. French deconstructionist Michel Foucault writes:

Illness is defined in relation to an average, a norm, a "pattern," and since the whole essence of the pathological resides within this departure: illness, it seems, is marginal by nature and relative to a culture only insofar as it is a form of behavior that is not integrated by that culture . . . mental illness takes its place among the possibilities that serve as a margin to the cultural reality of a social group.[16]

Mental Health: An Alternative Model

I would like to explore an alternative to how we conceptualize mental health. To consider such a conceptualization, we need to return to the basic element in our ontological structure: the need to make sense of the reality of the phenomenal world in which we live. This need to explain phenomena, including intrapsychic processes, results in the construction of explanations, from religion to science, to theories of personality, and the world of spirits and demons. Each construction, as explored in chapter two, leads to the formation of values. The scientific worldview values empirical thinking. Evangelical theology values witnessing and conversion. Zen values emptiness. Tao values nothingness. Buddha speaks of silence. Buddhists practice restraint. Hindus are greatly influenced by caste. Confucians honor ancestors. Formation of values determines categories of behavior. There is the good and the better. The better and the best. There are the bad, worse, and the worst. Bad behaviors. Good behaviors. Behaved better. Behaved badly. Dresses nicely. Dresses funny. Every value system presupposes a bell curve of perception and interpretation, of norms and standard deviation. I think she is good. I think he is bad. He is religious. He is unorthodox. Cultural worldviews form the context within which one is judged. There is the "is" and the "ought," success or failure. An individual experiences himself or herself within the context of societal norms and cultural values. The socialization process dictates one's self-identity. Here, too, one may experience integrity or conflicts. If an individual is not where he or she ought to be as culturally or religiously defined, then conflicts arise. Here lies the significance of religious beliefs or worldviews. How reality is defined impacts the way we experience ourselves. Conflict is conceptual. It is an interpretative process. An Adventist eating pork experiences much greater conflict than a Methodist eating bacon. A Hindu eating beef experiences much greater conflict than a Catholic eating a steak. A Jew eating a nonkosher food experiences much greater conflict than a Muslim eating meat. An American who does not talk to his dead ancestors does not understand the guilt of a Chinese who does not offer food to his ancestors. An Englishman does not understand the fear of Chinese people who forget to offer gifts to the spirits of the hungry ghosts. The list runs on. Inherent in every value system is the potential for conflict.

I believe that mental health is not defined by symptoms of depression, anxiety, or mania. Mental health depends largely on the experience of the self within the cultural context, its social norms or its religious beliefs. Conflict with culture emerges through basic emotions such as anger, sadness, or anxiety (fear). Prolonged conflict affects the chemical components that cause distressing symptoms. According to

Foucault, classical psychopathology presupposes abnormality as the cause of alienation, but he sees otherwise. Expressing Foucault's position on this issue, Hubert Dreyfus writes, "[S]ocial contradictions cause alienation, alienation causes defenses, defenses causes brain malfunction, and brain malfunction causes abnormal behavior."[17] Foucault states, "It is not because one is ill that one is alienated, but insofar as one is alienated that one is ill."[18]

The process leading to brain malfunction may be described as sensitization and kindling. Sensitization occurs when there may not be an obvious observable response to a stimulus. However, repetition of exposure to similar stimuli often leads to a full response. Further exposure to similar stimuli may result in a full response even though the intensity of the stimulus may not be as strong as the original stimulus. Over time, a full response may occur even in the absence of stimulus. When this automatic response takes place, kindling has occurred.[19] In explaining the mechanism of sensitization and kindling, psychiatrist Robert Hedaya writes:

Sensitization and kindling seem to occur via the process of neuromodulation.[20] In this process, psychosocial events (which, via the meaning assigned to them, may be stressful), and/or the affective episodes themselves, change the long-term activity or expression of the genes. The altered amounts and types of gene products can change the actual structure and function of the neuron. The alteration of reactivity of the individual neurons can occur via changed amounts and types of receptor protein, as well as alterations in the number of connections the cell has with other cells.[21]

If we see pathology as a result of conflicts emerging from one's perception and experience of reality, we are faced with the importance of religions and worldviews (scientific, psychological, etc.) in determining the state of mental health, and come to a deeper appreciation of Jung's position: "Among all my patients in the second half of life—that is to say, over thirty-five—there has not been one whose problem in the last resort was not that of finding a religious outlook on life. It is safe to say that every one of them fell ill because he had lost what the living religions of every age have given to their followers, and none of them has been really healed who did not regain his religious outlook."[22]

For this reason, the state of mental health is the understanding and experience of the self within one's context, which is shaped, formed, and informed by shared beliefs regarding life and reality. This experience of self takes into consideration the biological and genetic factors that may lead to a certain inclination or tendency in one's psychological makeup as well. This particular understanding of mental health seems to suggest that psychological theories are attempts to understand the reality of the human psyche, which comes with beliefs and values. The value of psychology seems to depend on its intentionality in the observation of the human psyche.

Spirituality, Integration, and Mental Health

If mental health is perceived as the experience of the self within the context of society's understanding of reality (which, in turn, promotes or prevents conflict within the self), then the healthiness of one's mental/emotional state depends on one's ability to deal effectively with conflicts. Contemporary psychotherapy resolves conflicts through assisting an individual in accomplishing desired goals. Numerous methods are employed, including setting realistic boundaries so that one may realize what is attainable and what is not, spelling out concrete goals, and defining manageable objectives that will ultimately lead to the desired goals. One way to resolve conflict is to empower a client to achieve his or her goals. The other method is to redefine those goals. If the conflict is intrapsychic, the client is encouraged to explore the unconscious and bring those elements into consciousness. Numerous sophisticated methodologies with complex conceptual and theoretical insights are used to address clients' conflicts, and this space is insufficient to describe all of them. I will only discuss the process of integration in the movement toward mental health and suggest that a mentally healthy individual does not necessarily represent an individual free from emotional distress or clinical symptoms.

A quick reference to a study by David Karp, previously mentioned in chapter four, may be of assistance here. Karp believes that chronically depressed patients make four transitions. The final transition, which is also a place of healing, occurs when an individual learns to accept his or her depression and decides to make the best of the situation. Numerous studies seem to support this movement. First, depressed individuals, even after successful treatment, still operate at one standard deviation lower than the norm. Second, approximately 50 percent of individuals who have recovered from depression will relapse within two years. Third, very few of those diagnosed with clinical depression experience a single episode. Speaking of depression, Thomas Moore writes:

Some feelings and thoughts seem to emerge only in a dark mood. Suppress the mood, and you will suppress those ideas and reflections. Depression may be as important a channel for valuable "negative" feelings, as expressions of affection are for the emotions of love. Feelings of love give birth naturally to gestures of attachment. In the same way, the void and grayness of depression evoke an awareness and articulation of thoughts otherwise hidden behind the screen of lighter moods. . . . Melancholy gives the soul an opportunity to express a side of its nature that is as valid as any other, but is hidden out of our distaste for its darkness and bitterness.[23]

Just like cancer patients experiencing spiritual renewal when they come to terms with their own mortality, individuals struggling with a sense of being different because of mental illness may discover healing through the process of integration. Healing takes place when they learn to embrace their nonbeing and heterogeneity; the conflict is resolved. Instead of nonbeing causing conflicting feelings, it becomes part of the self. As nonbeing becomes integrated into a person's self-understanding, conflicts no longer exist. Concluding his chapter "Honoring Symptoms as a Voice of the Soul," Moore writes: "I often think of this paradox as I sit with someone with tears in her eyes, searching for some way to deal with a death, a divorce, or a depression. It is a beast, this thing that stirs in the core of her being, but it is also the star of her innermost nature. We have to care for this suffering with extreme reverence so that, in our fear and anger at the beast, we do not overlook the star."[24]

Jung and Integration

One of the most fascinating models of integration is Jung's approach to the human psyche. Jung believes in the importance of embracing shadows in the process of nurturing mental health. Shadow symbolizes our dark side; unacceptable behaviors, thoughts, and feelings. Shadow includes the finiteness of humanity, such as shortcomings, weakness, and the emotional instability that we experience. It shows itself in archetypal figures that appear among the primitives in a wide range of personifications.

Shadow

The human psyche seeks to hide its shadow. It delineates the shadow from consciousness because of its inability to integrate and acknowledge the shadow as part of the self. This inability emerges from the sense that there is something "evil" about us that needs to be hidden. It is "evil" because it contains culturally undesirable attributes such as primal feelings, lust, aggression, hate, envy, and antisocial qualities. The shadow is not compatible with our ego image. In covering the shadow, we repress it. In repressing, it is not present in our consciousness.

According to Jung, what is suppressed cannot remain hidden. It has a voice and it speaks. It manifests itself. The shadow may be manifested in an inward, symbolic figure or projected to the external world. As a figure, it is embodied in the material of the unconscious as a dream figure personifying one or more of the dreamer's psychic qualities. In projection, one projects one or more of the latent unconscious traits upon someone in the environment who, because of certain qualities, is suited to the role. Projection often shows itself in a strong, obsessive, affective reaction, positive or negative, toward another person. This is especially true if the other person is relatively unknown to us. The person we cannot stand is often the one possessing a part of us that we are not able to acknowledge. Whether a dream figure or our own projections, we need to recognize that the qualities belong to us.

Shadow[25] has significant value and psychic energy. When it is unrecognized, it can be destructive to the soul. When it is recognized, it proves to be a gold mine. For this reason, it is important to confront our shadows. Confronting one's shadow is the first task in the process of individuation. To confront the shadow is to take a merciless and critical look at one's own nature. To take a merciless look at our shadow is to first experience our shadow through projection upon an object outside of us. This will hopefully lead to the ability to distinguish between ourselves and our shadow. This ability to distinguish will result in the ability to maintain an objective attitude toward our own personality.

Jung distinguishes two different forms of shadow. Personal shadow refers to the psychic features of the individual that are unlived from the beginning. Collective shadow belongs to the collective unconscious. Both forms are operative within the human psyche. The formation of the personal shadow begins in very early childhood, through interaction with parents and significant others in the immediate environment. Negative parental reactions toward a child's natural instincts can impair his or her capacity for expression in adult life. Children who are required to be nice, good, and never dirty, bad, or angry, learn from a very young age that to survive they must present only their positive side and repress instinctive urges. Very soon these children learn to hide these feelings from themselves, too. Developmentally, much of the personal shadow has been formed by the age of six or seven. This takes place not by what parents say but by how they behave and relate to the child.

Evil, Unconscious, and the Society

Shadow does not belong to individuals alone. It can be a part of nations and cultures. The United States saw its shadow in the assassination of John F. Kennedy. Germany witnessed its shadow during the regime of Hitler, and Japan saw its shadow during World War II. When one's shadow is unrecognized and remains in the unconscious, it has destructive power. For this reason, Jung believes that the world cannot reach a state of order unless this truth can generally be recognized. Unless an individual learns to deal with his/her shadow, the world cannot be a better place. This is so because, to Jung, wars, racial intolerance, and strife all stem from a concept of evil that is too incomplete and is not self-reflective.

The idea that coming to terms with one's shadow can have an effect on the totality of collective evil is one of the most socially significant concepts in Jung. It stems from a basic understanding of projection. We project onto others that which we are not able to integrate or come to terms with in ourselves. This takes place at the political level as well. That which has been repressed is being projected onto other persons or nations, so the tension we cannot stand within ourselves results in national strife and struggle. Jung's challenge to us is that we learn to withdraw our projections upon others and confront our own shadow.

Jung has been criticized for this theory by a number of people who see the process as self-centered. The concentration on the self through the process of psychological analysis has been criticized as antisocial, selfish, and self-absorbed. Jung has two answers to this criticism. First, he sees a person who deals with his or her shadow as fulfilling their primary responsibility to the community. We are not fit or equipped to fight the battles of society until we have begun to attack the evil within ourselves. To attack the evils of society without any comprehension of the evil in ourselves will only result in compounding the problem. The person who dives into the depths will find both God and the community. Second, we have been thrown into this chaos in the first place because we did not pay attention to our shadows. We have been thrown off balance because we were one-sided. It's time to pay attention to our souls and learn to deal with the shadow figures in them.

Spirituality, Integration, and Mental Health

For Boisen and many who share dark emotions and have journeyed into the abyss, spirituality is the intense quest to make sense of the tortured soul, to find meaning in chaos, and to make sense of the senseless. It is a process of examining the place of emptiness, alienation, obsession, unspeakable sadness, and pain in one's life. Could this pain mean something or am I suffering for nothing? The process of integration brings about a sense of comfort with oneself, with one's vulnerability, with one's pain and limitations. It is about the courage to accept and learn to deal effectively with one's vulnerability. It is the self that comes to terms with itself or, as Gerald May has wisely stated, "It all, just simply, is."[26] Spirituality is an invitation to return to one's self as it is. It is the path that leads home. Spirituality offers the promise that it is all right to let go because there is Something much bigger that supports and sustains us.

CHAPTER SEVEN

Integration | The Case of Søren Kierkegaard

There was once a father and a son. A son is like a mirror in which the father beholds himself, and for the son the father too is like a mirror in which he beholds himself in the time to come. However, they rarely regarded one another in this way, for their daily intercourse was characterized by the cheerfulness of gay and lively conversation. It happened only a few times that the father came to a stop, stood before the son with a sorrowful countenance, looked at him steadily and said: "Poor child, you are going into a quiet despair." True as this saying was, nothing was ever said to indicate how it was to be understood. And the father believed that he was to blame for the son's melancholy, and the son believed that he was the occasion of the father's sorrow—but they never exchanged a word on this subject.

–Søren Kierkegaard, "The Quiet Despair"[1]

Søren Aabye Kierkegaard was born on May 5, 1813, in Copenhagen, Denmark. He spent his whole life in Copenhagen. He died there on November 4, 1855, and was buried in the family plot.[2] To understand his psyche, one needs to review his past in relation to his father, Michael Kierkegaard, who Kierkegaard believed had imparted to him the "conception of the divine father-love, the one unshakable thing in life, the true Archimedean point."[3]

Father

Michael Kierkegaard was born in the desolate heath of West Jutland to a family of nine children. At a very young age, while believing that he was "condemned to a life of poverty and obscurity," he was chosen by his uncle, Niels Andersen Seding, to go to Copenhagen, where he established a small business as a hosier. Michael Kierkegaard became prosperous[4] at a very young age and retired[5] from active life at the age of forty, leaving his nephew, Michael Andersen Kierkegaard, to run the business.

On April 26, 1797, Michael Kierkegaard married his second wife, Ane Sorendatter Lund (the servant girl who served the family before his first wife passed away). It is interesting to note that their first child, Maren Kirsten, was born on September 7, 1797, exactly four months and eleven days after the marriage. This incident had a great impact upon Michael's personal integrity as a religious man and on Søren later in his life, since he looked up to his father as a model of morality. Nicoline Christine, Petrea Severine, and Peter Christian were born in the course of the next eight years. Søren Michael was born in 1807 and Niels Andreas was born two years after. When Michael Kierkegaard was fifty-one and Ane Sorendatter was forty-five, Søren Aabye Kierkegaard was born, the last of the seven children.

Michael was a very religious person and brought up all his children in the fear of God.[6] He had a very keen mind and often engaged in philosophical debates. Michael was also very melancholic, which affected all his children, particularly Søren Aabye Kierkegaard.[7] Whether his melancholy was inherited or otherwise, there is no way of knowing. We do know that most of his children were physically frail (suggested by their early deaths) and that there was a family history of psychic instability. Peter Christian was compelled to resign from his office as bishop when he came close to insanity. Peter's son was confined to an asylum and was yet witty enough to say, "My uncle was Either/Or, my father is Both/And, and I am Neither/Nor." Another of Søren's nephews had several insanity attacks and one of them committed suicide.

Besides having a history of psychic instability, a story was told that one day as a shepherd boy in Jutland, Michael Kierkegaard, suffering much from hunger, cold, and loneliness, stood upon a hummock, lifted his hands to heaven, and cursed the Lord God for being so hard-hearted as to let a helpless, innocent child suffer so much without coming to his aid. When blessings came through his prosperity, Michael realized that he had cursed the true God and was aware of the depth of his sin. It was the awareness of this curse that led him to bring up his children in a strict religious atmosphere. This story was supposedly related to Søren in full just before his father's death.[8] And it was around this period, too, that Søren learned of his father's sensuality. These events were like an "earthquake" in Søren's life.

Søren Kierkegaard

Childhood

Kierkegaard describes his childhood as half child-play, half God in the heart. The religious education imparted by his father made a deep impression upon him and yet he was playful as a child. Even then, he was sharp with his words and polemical. This earned him rebukes from his teachers and a bloody nose from a bigger playmate. His schoolmates described him as "a regular wild cat." Apparently, his "play" was not socially "conformed." He was nicknamed "Choirboy" because of his dress (it resembled the costume in charity schools).

Physically, Søren was a very frail child, and it was this, he believed, that would cause his early death. A marked curvature of the spine was caused by a fall from a tree in early childhood. Spinal trouble was the hospital diagnosis.[9] Physical inferiority plagued his family. Two of his siblings died before he was nine and a few years later three died in quick succession. This caused him acute distress throughout his life, and he described his body as "a disproportion between my soul and my body." In a journal entry, he described his childhood:

I was already an old man when I was born. . . . Delicate, slender, and weak, deprived of almost every condition for holding my own with other boys, or even for passing as a complete human being in comparison with others; melancholy, sick in soul, in many ways profoundly unfortunate, one thing I had: an eminently shrewd wit, given me presumably in order that I might not be defenseless. . . . I am in the deepest sense an unfortunate individual who has from the earliest age been nailed fast to one suffering or another, to the very verge of insanity.[10]

Youth

At the age of seventeen, he started his theological education, according to his father's wishes. He was a diligent and brilliant student. Three years later, he started his journal.[11] It was around this time that his sister, Nicoline Christine, died at the age of thirty-three while giving birth to a stillborn baby. A year later, his brother, Niels Andreas, died at the age of twenty-five. These deaths were keenly felt by Søren.

At twenty-two, Søren learned of his father's curse—the curse that caused Michael to live in anxious dread and to believe that his children were condemned to the silence of despair—the reason he took on the sternest requirements of Christianity. Søren also learned that the man he revered as an example of morality had violated his mother when she was a virgin, while she was a servant-maid.[12] Søren felt the anger of God keenly. In his *Concept of Dread*, in view of the shattering experience of learning the truth about his father, he wrote, "Dread [*Angst*] is not sudden like a dart, but slowly bores its way into the heart."[13]

It was around this period that Søren felt that he was not living a complete human life. He reflected: "What I really need is to become clear in my own mind what I must do, not what I must know. . . . The important thing is to understand what I am destined for, to perceive what the Deity wants me to do: the point is to find that which is truth for me, to find that idea for which I am ready to live and die."[14] This idea was later developed into his concept of "truth as subjectivity."

The Great Earthquake

The earthquake experience caused great distress in Søren's life and influenced his development in the ensuing months, a time he described as the "shipwreck of freedom." "All sin begins with fear," Søren wrote in 1837, and upon reflection in May 1843, he wrote: "It was dread that caused me to go astray." His activities at the time were partly influenced by the medieval legends of Faust and Don Juan. Faust in particular invites the reader to "pass through every vice just to acquire experience of life."[15] From Don Juan, Søren learned sensuality, and a time of defiance began. "In order to will in despair to be oneself there must be consciousness of the infinite self. This infinite self, however, is really only the abstractest form, the abstractest possibility of the self, and it is this self the man despairingly wills to be, detaching the self from every relation to that Power which posited it."[16] But Søren did not realize that his defiance could lead to despair. He believed himself to be "uncommonly erotic," "uncommon" because of his rare sense of shame. He was more distressed by impure suggestions of sensuality than are most men. In April, Søren had fallen very low. The entry suggests that he was often drunk and frequently thought of suicide.[17] It is generally agreed that his sexual "fall" was in the month of May.[18] Søren attributed this fall to "dread": "my lusts and excesses—which yet perhaps in God's sight were not so atrocious, for indeed it was dread which caused me to go astray."

From this entry, we learn that Søren made a moral resolution, but there were occasions of relapse, as we see in his record on June 12, 1836: "Reformation goes slowly. As Franz Baader justly remarked, one must retrace the same path by which one went."[19] Lowrie's description of Søren during this period is worth considering: "During this period of frequent drunkenness and constant intellectual inebriation he often felt that he was on the verge of madness."[20] What accentuated his "dread" was the fact that he was still living in the same house as his father, the man who was the tower of morality; the man who had cursed God and violated a virgin.

Groping His Way Back

On June 4, Søren wrote: "I have just come from a party of which I was the soul: witticism flowed from my mouth, all laughed and admired me, but I went . . . and wanted to shoot myself." This suicidal statement was triggered by a comment Poul Moller made at the party to Søren: "You are so polemicalized through and through that it is perfectly terrible."[21] Till the end of his life, Søren remembered this comment, which he described as "the great awakening." It had a great impact on him because through it he realized that his defiance against God was caused by his polemical nature. It was around this time that he started reading George Hamann. Hamann's quote from Hume's *Inquiry Concerning the Human Understanding* is worth repeating here: "Mere reason is not sufficient to convince us of its veracity: and whoever is moved by Faith to assent to it, is conscious of a continued miracle in his own person, which subverts all the principles of his understanding, and gives him a determination to believe what is most contrary to custom and experience."[22] It was the realization of the demonic nature of his "polemic" and that "faith transcends reason" that later led to Søren's conversion experience.

On his twenty-fifth birthday, his father confessed to him the sin he had committed, suspecting that perhaps it was Søren's discovery of his misconduct that had driven his son away from home and God. It is believed that Søren was moved on this occasion to ask for his father's forgiveness. According to Lowrie, "in returning to his father S.K. returned to God."[23] During this time Søren realized he had repeated his father's sin, which inspired him to spend his life doing penance.[24] Fifteen days after his twenty-fifth birthday, he recorded this entry (May 19, 10:30 a.m.):

There is such a thing as an indescribable joy which glows through us as unaccountably as the Apostle's outburst is unexpected: 'Rejoice, and again I say, Rejoice!'—Not a joy over this or that, but full jubilation, 'with hearts, and souls, and voices': 'I rejoice over my joy, of, in, by, at, on, through, with my joy'—a heavenly refrain, which cuts short, as it were, our ordinary song; a joy which cools and refreshes like a breeze, a gust of the trade wind which blows from the Grove of Mamre to the eternal mansions.[25]

Regina

Kierkegaard's love for Regina Olsen was "love at first sight." About three years after he met her, he proposed, and on September 10, 1840, they were engaged. In October of 1841, he broke the engagement and fled to Berlin.[26] But Regina was always in his thoughts and heart to the very last day of his life. His niece describes his condition after he broke the engagement: "He looked terribly upset and instead of his usual teasing, he kissed me so gently on the hair that I was touched to the heart. A moment later, when he was waiting to talk to us, he burst into violent weeping, and without really knowing what there was to weep about." Reflecting on that autumn day, he later wrote: "When I left her I chose death."[27]

Cloister

In the years following his breakup with Regina, Søren began to withdraw further and further from the world. Yet through this withdrawal, he became engaged once again through his writings. Between 1842 and 1846 he wrote *Either/Or, Two Edifying Discourses, Four Edifying Discourses, Fear and Trembling, Repetition, Three Edifying Discourses,*

Philosophical Fragments, The Concept of Dread, Prefaces, Three Discourses on Imagined Occasions, Stages on Life's Way, and *Concluding Unscientific Postscript.*

His solitude was made possible by the fortune his father had left him. Although his accounts showed his generous spending habits (on himself), he did not spend his money carelessly, "but used it up with great deliberation to construct the 'cloister' in which he could work fruitfully, without interruption or distraction."[28] In 1850, he wrote, "[B]ut for my extravagance, I would never have been able to work on such a scale."[29]

Corsair[30]

Søren's attacks on the newspaper *Corsair* had unpleasant consequences. The paper started with subtle attacks that soon became more obvious and acidic. Before long, every issue of the *Corsair* carried something spiteful on Kierkegaard.

Besides articles there were drawings that caricatured Kierkegaard's peculiarities—his bent back and thin legs, his perennial walking stick or umbrella, his crablike gait, his uneven trousers, one leg shorter than the other. The joke about the trousers caught the public imagination. Small children would run up to him and stare at his pants, and once he sat down in church only to find two young men studying his legs and mocking him. Even his tailor began to wish that Kierkegaard would take his business elsewhere. Corsair embroidered the joke with an announcement on February 19 that "the author of *Either/Or*, Mr. Victor Eremita, won a prize at the Industrial Union for an essay on the manufacture of clothing in Denmark. The motto to the essay was as follows: 'We all know from experience that either the two legs of trousers are equally long, or that one is longer than the other.'"[31]

Kierkegaard's usual enjoyable walk down the street, conversing with servant girls and cab drivers, and observing the everyday life of everyday people, was taken from him. He continued to walk, but he no longer experienced the same pleasure. He saw this as God's call for sacrifice. He was "God's gift" to his people. Through God's providence, he would lead the Danish people to Christianity; his was a divinely sanctioned martyrdom.

Metamorphosis

On August 16, 1847, Kierkegaard wrote in his journal:

I feel now impelled to come to myself in a deeper sense, by coming closer to God in the understanding of myself. I must remain on the spot and be renewed inwardly. . . . *I must try to get a better hold upon my melancholy* [my italics]. . . . There is something stirring in me which indicates a *metamorphosis* [my italics]. Precisely for this reason I did not dare to take the trip to Berlin—for that would be to produce an abortion. I shall therefore keep quiet, not work too hard, yea, hardly at all, not begin a new book, but try to come to myself, *to think thoroughly the thought of my melancholy together with God on the spot.* In that way my melancholy may be relieved and Christianity come closer to me.[32]

The year 1848 was a very important year in his life. Professor Hirsch writes: "the year 1848 represents the climax of Kierkegaard's intellectual productiveness. . . . *The Sickness unto Death* and *Training in Christianity* (his two masterpieces as a Christian author) and *The Point of View*."[33] This productivity reflects a very important religious experience in his life: the discovery of faith, faith in the forgiveness and forgetfulness of God. On April 19, 1848, he wrote: "My whole nature is changed. My close reserve, my introversion, is broken—I must speak. Great God, give me grace!" About a week later, he recorded: "[W]hat marvelous boldness of faith is involved in believing that the sin is entirely forgotten, so that the memory of it has nothing alarming about it, thus truly believing oneself into being a new man, so that one can scarcely recognize oneself again."[34]

With this new disposition, Kierkegaard wrote: "[A] hope has awakened in my soul that God may desire to resolve the fundamental misery of my being. That is to say, now I am in faith in the profoundest sense."[35] This experience had a great impact upon his life.[36] Although he experienced frequent relapses[37] and never actualized his hope "to resolve the fundamental misery of [his] being," it nevertheless was a "radical cure" for him and a necessary step toward a greater discovery of God's call.

In 1852, Kierkegaard came to the realization that "melancholy" was his calling, that he was called to be different and, in being different, to stand as a witness for truth. Kierkegaard believed that his orientation gave him insight into Christianity. On June 19, 1852, he wrote in his journal:

The polemical craft which is my natural characteristic and is inseparable from my very being is here again in place. . . . O my God, how clearly it now all stands out before me, how endlessly much has already been done for me. It is not difference that I must pray myself out of, that is not the task, but alas, I shall never know security, which consists in being like others. No, I remain different. . . . I have suffered so very much in the past year and had to consider everything so seriously that doubtless I am a good deal changed. . . . I feel peaceful and happy, perhaps more definitely so and with a more tranquil confidence than in 1848.[58]

From this time on, there were no relapses, "no symptom of the hesitation which is so painful a feature of the earlier journals." Kierkegaard knew what he was called to do, and from this period on, he launched his attack on the church. This he did as a witness to the truth, a little pinch of spice.[59]

Death

On October 2, 1855, Kierkegaard fell unconscious on the street. He was carried to Frederik's Hospital and, as he entered, he said, "I've come here to die." Kierkegaard was sent to Dr. Seligmann Trier's ward where he received some of the best treatment available at the time. He was diagnosed with staphylococcus infection.[40] On November 18, 1855, forty days after he was admitted, he died.

Spirituality, Theology, and Integration in the Life of Kierkegaard

In reading about Kierkegaard's life and theological development along with the *Diagnostic Statistical Manual* (DSM-IV) and other materials on depression and anxiety, I cannot help but notice the interplay between chemistry and theology. It seems as though Kierkegaard's theological reflections were an attempt at coping or dealing with anxiety and depression. In his personal life, Kierkegaard constantly struggled with "something ghostly" about himself, something unreal. In 1849, the year *The Sickness Unto Death* was published, he wrote: "I was always, always outside myself." In his theological writings, we see the dialectic between ideality and actuality. Kierkegaard was constantly searching for the "actual." In *The Concept of Anxiety*, he sought the actualization of ideality. From an ethical point of view, we may see this search as a typical ethical struggle between the "is" and the "ought." But seeing that this concept appeared in *The Concept of Anxiety,* and that he personally struggled with anxiety, the connection between derealization and his theological proposition of ideality and actuality becomes a real possibility.[41]

Assuming that the above diagnosis is correct, the following theological statement from *The Sickness Unto Death* is clarified:

So to be sick unto death is, not to be able to die—yet not as though there were hope of life; no, the hopelessness in this case is that even the last hope, death, is not available. When death is the greatest danger, one hopes for life; but when one becomes acquainted with an even more dreadful danger, one hopes for death. So when the danger is so great that death has become one's hope, despair is the disconsolateness of not being able to die.

It is in this last sense that despair is the sickness unto death, this agonizing contradiction, this sickness in the self, everlastingly to die, to die and yet not to die, to die the death. For dying means that it is all over, but dying the death means to live to experience death.[42]

This theological statement seems to reflect Kierkegaard's personal struggle with melancholy; it is a theological construct interpreting his existential struggle. Perhaps it was not his anxiety alone that affected his theology, but the reverse may also be true. Kierkegaard's first major depressive episode was caused by his theological interpretation of his father's sin. In 1850, reflecting on his childhood years, he wrote:

The greatest danger is not that his father or tutor should be a free-thinker, not even his being a hypocrite. No, the danger lies in his being a pious, God-fearing man, and in the child being convinced thereof, but that he should nevertheless notice that deep in his soul there lies hidden an unrest which, consequently, not even the fear of God and piety could calm. The danger is that the child in that situation is almost provoked to draw a conclusion about God, that God is not infinite love.[43]

Commenting on Kierkegaard's "earthquake experience," Lowrie writes: "The sudden confirmation of his father's guilt was the 'frightful upheaval' which imposed upon Søren a new infallible rule for interpreting all the 'phenomena' which had aroused his suspicion."[44] No wonder Kierkegaard saw himself as the "object of the fury of the angry gods." His theology intensified his interpretation of events, causing him the great distress that led to his "astray" experience and, ultimately, to his first major depressive episode.

It is also interesting that the turning points in his life started with two theological concepts: the leap of faith, which allows one to accept that God forgives and forgets, and, secondly, his acceptance of life as it is. Kierkegaard's experience of forgiveness through faith came in 1848, when he described "belief in the forgiveness of sins" as the belief "that here in time the sin is forgotten by God, that it is really true that God forgets."[45] And in 1852, he wrote, "Then came 1848. I was lifted up to a height which I had never before known, and perfectly understood myself in what had gone before, and the past."[46] In 1852, Kierkegaard came to accept his God-given destiny, his heterogeneity. He was to be different; he was called to melancholy. Kierkegaard realized that it was through this "heterogeneity" that he was to serve God. Although the thorn in his flesh never left, it did not bother him but empowered him for his service to God. On June 19, 1852, he wrote: "I feel peaceful and happy, perhaps more definitely so and with a more tranquil confidence than in 1848."[47]

From the perspective of integration, Kierkegaard's existential struggle led him ultimately to accept his melancholia as his destiny, as the place from which he could contribute to society. Viewing his theology from an existential perspective (his personal struggle with melancholia and anxiety) helps us understand that, while using theology as a tool to cope, he found peace in a theology that embraced nonbeing, the negatives in life. It would be reasonable to believe that Kierkegaard found peace when his theology permitted full acceptance of his own heterogeneity.

CHAPTER EIGHT

Spiritual Assessment

The North Wind and the Sun were having an argument as to who was the stronger. The Sun said, "I know a way to settle the argument. Do you see that man coming down the road? Whichever one of us makes him take off his coat will be reckoned the stronger." The North Wind agreed. The Sun hid behind a cloud while the North Wind whistled and the man shivered. It roared and raged and sent icy blasts against the man. But the harder the wind blew, the closer the man wrapped his coat about him. Then the Sun had a turn. The Sun shone gently and the man unbuttoned his coat. Then the Sun covered the whole earth with warmth and within a few minutes the man was so hot he took off his coat.

—Aesop's Fable[1]

Development is a natural process we all go through. It assumes that, under normal circumstances, people naturally make a transition toward greater maturity and greater appreciation of complexity. The idea of spiritual growth is based on the same assumption. However, the way we conceptualize spiritual maturity is diverse. There are many ideal stages proposed by various religious traditions, denominations, and theorists. Spiritual goals are based on reality as defined and perceived by various traditions influenced by cultural, historic, socioeconomic, and environmental factors, so there are various methods of assessment.[2] Spiritual assessment never assumes a neutral position. It comes with theological assumptions. One's spirituality may be judged by one's moral character, one's response to injustice, one's piety, one's engagement in religious activities, one's eagerness to share one's faith, and even one's choice of food. I grew up in a church where spirituality was monitored through church engagement, frequency of prayer, punctilious behavioral compliance, voraciousness in Bible reading, passion in witnessing, and the correspondence of personal beliefs to one's denominational statements. There is no one way to define spiritual growth and maturity. It is important for caregivers to recognize that there are multiple modalities of spiritual growth. And growth is always defined by its assumptions or truth-claims. The process of spiritual assessment must be conscious of the assumptions under which it operates.

My approach to spiritual assessment assumes that spirituality is movement toward the integration of nonbeing, the need to see meaning even in the midst of pain, suffering, and mortality, while God remains a comfort through difficult times. This type of transition is possible for people who are able to embrace paradoxes and ambiguities. Assuming absolutes in theological constructions disengages the process. Certainty of theological knowledge leaves no room for ambiguity. The theological implication of transitional spirituality is a God who is weak and powerless, as Bonhoeffer stated. "The Bible directs man to God's powerlessness and suffering; only the suffering God can help."[3] In explaining this concept, he writes, "It is only by living completely in this world that one learns to have faith. . . . By this-worldliness-I mean living unreservedly in life's duties, problems, successes and failures, experiences and perplexities. In so doing we throw ourselves completely into the arms of God, taking seriously, not our own sufferings, but those of God in the world—watching with Christ in Gethsemane."[4]

Numerous theologians and religious writers have expressed this transition into a more mystical understanding of God. James Fowler describes conjunctive faith: "Alive to paradox and the truth in apparent contradictions, this stage strives to unify opposites in mind and experience. It generates and maintains vulnerability to the strange truths of those who are 'Other.' Ready for closeness to that which is different and threatening to self and outlook (including new depths of experience in spirituality and religious revelation)."[5]

> Lao Tzu tells us the mystery of the Real:
> The Tao that can be told

is not the eternal Tao.
The name that can be named
is not the eternal Name.

The unnamable is the eternally real.
Naming is the origin
of all particular things.[6]

Chuang Tzu is in agreement when, in *The Inner Chapters*, he writes: "Therefore understanding that rests in what it does not understand is the finest. Who can understand discriminations that are not spoken, the Way that is not a way? If he can understand this, he may be called the Reservoir of Heaven. Pour into it and it is never full, dip from it and it never runs dry, and yet it does not know where the supply comes from."[7]

When Buddha's disciples asked him a question pertaining to the existence of God, Buddha replied with silence and a smile. Silence may be or may be not a denial of God, but it suggests a sense of mystery. The smile is an invitation to embrace this mystery and, through validating it, affirm it by living as meaningfully and productively as we possibly can.[8] Speaking of the place of silence in the search for the sacred, Krishnamurti suggests: "That which is holy, that which is sacred, which is truth, can only be when there is complete silence. . . . Out of that immense silence there is that which is sacred."[9]

Spiritual growth in Hinduism is also movement, toward the stage of *sanyasin*,[10] a person unharmed by the world yet living in the world. The *sanyasin* is a person who has come to understand the world beyond the seen, and life beyond senses, one who has a sense of bliss. Swami Vevekananda describes a *sanyasin* in a song:

Heed then no more how body lives or goes,
Its task is done. Let Karma float it down;
Let one put garlands on, another kick
This frame; say naught. No praise or blame can be
Where praiser praised, and blamer blamed are one.
Thus be thou calm, Sannyasin bold! Say—
"Om Tat Sat, Om!"[11]

Religious traditions from ancient time realize the impact spiritual growth and development have on us, on how we cope and deal with life's pain and gain, humor and tragedy, sorrow and laughter. The place of God or the sacred in one's life determines the quality of one's life. Based on this assumption regarding human spiritual development, I propose the following approach to spiritual assessment for caregivers who recognize the importance of the role of spirituality in the healing process, and who are involved in caring for people in the midst of life's turmoil and tragedy.

Spiritual Assessment

There are numerous helpful modalities of spiritual assessment that can be utilized by caregivers who wish to fine-tune their skills. Harold Koenig suggests four questions that we should pay special attention to while taking a spiritual history: Is religion or spirituality being employed as a method of coping with illness? Does the patient have a supportive spiritual community? Are there spiritual questions that are of concern to the patient? Are there spiritual beliefs that may affect medical care?[12]

Richard L. Gorsuch and William R. Miller propose that the following questions could be incorporated during the process of clinical interviews: Do you currently practice your religion? Do you believe in God or a Higher Power? Are there certain practices that you engage in on a regular basis? In assessing a sense of meaning, they suggest we ask: What is important to you and what gives you meaning and purpose in life?[13] These questions are helpful as we consider spiritual assessment. The following approach is based primarily on the model of integration, seeking to learn the extent to which a person has incorporated nonbeing into his or her system of meaning.

Meaning of Pain

Based on the assumption that there is an ontological drive to make sense of life, particularly in the presence of tragedy, individuals face the task of redefining the meaning of their existence within the reality of the threat of nonbeing. The natural question emerging from this process is the question "Why?" Why must this thing happen to me? What good does it do for me? How can there be any sense to such a terrible thing? The struggle with this question itself is a strong indication that integration has not taken place. The question has not been answered. There is still a strong feeling that this tragedy is senseless and there seems to be no possible explanation that can be reasonable enough. "It just does not make sense." A person's existential struggle with the question of purpose and meaning when confronted with tragedy is often a good indication that his or her worldview is not able to accommodate pain, suffering, and mortality at the existential level.[14]

Questions that can be used to assess the meaning assigned to suffering and mortality are: Have you ever asked God why this thing is happening? Do you struggle with the "Why" question? Do you ever wonder if there is any purpose in this? Do you know why this is happening to you?

God and Miracles

Another theological indication is the movement toward the supernatural, the miraculous intervention. This may be indicated through religious language. "I know God will save me." "I know God is capable of removing this cancer." "I'm praying for a miracle to happen." "I really believe in miracles." It is not uncommon for individuals who may, at the cognitive level, embrace the view that pain, suffering, and mortality are a part of life, to believe in a God of miraculous intervention when they are actually confronting the reality of their mortality existentially. Evoking God for a miraculous intervention reflects a patient's attempt to retain his or her previous existential view of reality as a source of meaning. William A. Fintel and Gerald R. McDermott recount the story of Floyd, whose son, Jimmy, was diagnosed with leukemia: "Though Jimmy does not fully understand the dangers of this cancer, Floyd does. Right now, therefore, Floyd is the one who's really suffering. And the question that is tormenting Floyd is the same question that millions of believers have asked for centuries: If God is all-good and all-powerful, why would he permit a terrible disease like cancer?"[15]

Floyd's struggle and the question raised reflect his intense desire to make sense of the suffering and mortality which do not seem to fit his system of meaning.

Questions that may be relevant in assessing theological positions include: Where is God in your struggle? Do you think about God while you are going through this? How do you think God is involved with your life as you face this illness?

Fantasy

A twelve-year-old girl who lives with her mom and stepfather wrote me a story during one of our counseling sessions.

Once upon a time there was a prince. He wished that he would meet the right woman one day. But his father didn't want him to find the right girl. He wanted him to find the prettiest girl. One day his father saw the prettiest girl he had ever seen in the whole entire world. He tried to stop her but a truck passed by and he lost her. The next few days that was all he could think about. One day the father went out and saw the girl again but this time he met her and took her to the palace. The prince met her and wanted to get to know her so they went to dinner and the girl told the prince that she wasn't as pretty as she looked. He told her that that wasn't what mattered to him. That night he kissed her and she turned into a poor slave girl like she was before. She told him about the spell that would break after her first kiss. They got married. The end.

After we read the story she said that when she grew up she would find a very good-looking and nice man. Someone who would love her no matter how bad she behaved at times; someone who would always be there for her. They would be really in love, get married, have children, and live together happily ever after. Then she added, "I know it's just a fantasy. But I like fantasy."

The language of fantasy is another indicator of a compliation of spiritual movement. Fantasy speaks beyond the present reality. Fantasy suggests a patient is unable to deal with the immense pain of the reality confronting him or her. In fantasy, a terminally ill patient may speak of his or her ten-year goals, a physically handicapped person may speak of imminent recovery when he or she will be physically active, or a diabetic patient plans a big feast. Speaking of fantasy, Ethel Person writes, "Perhaps most important of all, daydreaming lends solace in sorrow and pain. Fantasizing a happier future may permit us to bear an untenable present rather than be overwhelmed by depression and feelings of hopelessness."[16]

Possible questions to ask the patient who is fantasizing include:

What is your understanding of your illness and its impact on your life? When you think about the future, what comes to mind?

Respecting Diversity

Perhaps the most crucial thing in spiritual assessment is to remain open to various possibilities. Constructs are mere guides. What is important is to seek an understanding of how individuals assign meaning to the tragic events they are going through and to be willing to modify our constructs of spiritual growth and development. Spirituality is not something that can be placed in a neatly designed construct. Spirituality adapts itself through the contour of one's internal psychological structure, environment, culture, history, and social context. Caregivers must always remain open and be willing to learn. In fact, spiritual assessment is first and foremost an attitude of learning so that we may be more effective in assisting others. A caregiver does not step into a patient's room as an expert who seeks to assess in order to offer prescriptions for the soul. On the other hand, a caregiver does come in with a willingness to learn from and about the patient, and with a desire to understand what role, if any, spirituality plays in the patient's quest for meaning when he or she is faced with real and existentially painful tragedy.

Acknowledging Complexity: Respecting the Sacred

From a theological perspective, our approach to the understanding of human souls needs to emerge from our acknowledgement of the sacredness of others. Assessment here is not about assessing in order to prescribe; it is about coming to a deeper sense of appreciation and respect for the divine elements in those we are ministering to, acknowledging the complexity and the sacred in others. Perhaps it is most appropriate to summarize this chapter reflecting on Kosuke Koyama's interpretation of the parable of the wind and the sun. The North Wind and the Sun argued about who was the stronger of the two and, to settle the argument, they decided that whoever could get the man to take off his coat would be the winner. The North Wind started blowing and the man wrapped himself up. The harder the North Wind blew, the tighter the man held on to his coat. Then the Sun shown gently and the man started to unbutton his coat. When the Sun increased its warmth, the man took off his coat. Koyama's theological interpretation of this parable seems quite appropriate for caregivers: "Let me summarize the difference between the North Wind and the Sun. It is this: the former was interested first in the coat and then in the man, while the latter saw the man first then the coat. That is to say, the former ignored the truth that man is not that simple—man is a puzzle—whereas the later recognized and respected man's dignity and self-determination."[17]

It is a theological necessity, argues Koyama, that we acknowledge the complexity and mystery that is human.

The North Wind view of life ignores all this mysterious depth of man. It is thus bound to be a superficial understanding of man's life. We cannot and must not approach man by "blowing." "Blowing" is an attack upon the dignity of man, and it is also an insult upon man's amazing inner spiritual quality. Let us remain ever amazed at the tremendously intricate mind and spirituality of man! Let man come first, then the coat! Not the North Wind view of life but the Sun view of life. We all know that a man wears a coat; the coat cannot wear the man![18]

CHAPTER NINE

Spiritual Care

All who serve, serve life. What we serve is something worthy of our attention, of the commitment of our time and our lives. Service is not about fixing life, outwitting life, manipulating life, controlling life, or struggling to gain mastery over life. When we serve, we discover that life is holy.

—Rachel Naomi Remen[1]

Spiritual care is the process of enabling individuals to modify their systems of meaning in order to existentially integrate nonbeing into their understanding of life and reality. It is the art of being there in such a way as to facilitate the transitional process for those going through trauma. The primary task of spiritual caregivers is to enter the world of paradox that reflects the nature of the soul. One of the most essential processes in helping someone move forward is to go backward, to seemingly negate the very goal we wish to achieve. In this case, caring requires that we give up the desire to help an individual move forward and cease attempting to propel them into transition. Caring is being fully where the person is. Upon entering this process, it is helpful for spiritual caregivers to be aware of certain essential concepts.

Spiritual Journey

The journey toward this transition is something that an individual who faces chronic illness or trauma has to make by him- or herself. If an individual has not made the transition, there is nothing the caregiver can do about it except respect that fact. The task of the caregiver is not to try to move a person from point A to point B. People need to make this journey by themselves, in their own way. If their way takes them in a circular or regressive process, then it is somehow important for them to make the journey that way.

The path may not be a linear, prescriptive one, but each step of it is sacred, though its course may appear pathological to caregivers. As Friedrich Nietzsche put it, "In this world there is one unique path which no one but you may walk. Where does it lead? Do not ask, take it."[2] A chaplain once related the story of a male patient he visited. The man had just completed his undergraduate degree and was ready to start working when an auto accident took his wife and children from him, and he was left a paraplegic. During the initial chaplain's visit, the patient told the chaplain that his faith was strong, that God was good to him, and that everything would turn out all right. But that was just the beginning of many visits, as the chaplain walked with the patient through intense anger toward God, enormous grief, and finally, to healing, where God remained with him in his brokenness, offering hope for the future.

This transitional process needs to be existential in nature. How it is to be accomplished cannot be prescribed. Each individual has to live through it and experience it in all its manifestations. Every aspect of a person's life has to interact fully with this occurrence. Patients have to make sense of their crisis in relation to their psyche, past history, social relations, and theology. The journey has to be experienced as the path unfolds. There is no "point" to get to, no "place" to arrive at; the path is wherever the individual is. It is sacred. The journey is essential and cannot be quickened, prescribed, or forced to happen. It goes where it wants to go.

Spiritual Care

The art of providing spiritual care is to go with patients wherever their journey takes them. It is just to be there. "To be there" is to be a presence that does not seek to alter, fix, or prescribe a way of being. James Dittes, professor of pastoral care and counseling at Yale Divinity School, suggests the role of witness, witness to the lives of others in all their facets. In his book, *Pastoral Counseling: The Basics*, he states, "Fundamentally, the pastoral counselor does not try to 'do' anything and is not struggling to make something happen, to make repairs, or to make changes. The intent of pastoral counseling is more profound than that. The pastoral counselor witnesses."[3]

Another metaphor for spiritual care is hospitality. Stephen Muse of the Pastoral Institute believes that true psychotherapy is an invitation to extend hospitality to strangers. This process is reciprocal in nature. The people we pay attention to in therapy sessions invite us into the sacred tents of their lives where hidden treasures are kept. Often, new therapists are too eager to fix, probe, and analyze. But with maturity, we become quieter and begin to notice others more fully. "We learn that much of life involves suffering we can do nothing to alleviate. Rather, it is the human suffering which, rightly engaged, produces maturity and strength of character."[4] In *Care of the Soul*, Thomas Moore makes a distinction between the care for and cure of the soul. Caring for the soul, he states, "isn't about curing, fixing, changing, adjusting or making healthy, and it isn't about some idea of perfection or even improvement. It doesn't look to the future for an ideal, trouble-free existence. Rather, it remains patiently in the present, close to life as it presents itself day by day, and yet at the same time mindful of religion and spirituality."[5]

To be there for others is to permit them to stay right where they are in the midst of their depression, anger, frustration, doubt, fear, sadness, denial, fantasy, or tears. It is the gift of presence. Being there is remaining with them in all aspects of their experience, allowing them the space to be in touch with the depths of their pain. To remain with them in their depression is not attempting to get them to snap out of it. To remain with them in their anger is not letting their anger push us away from them. To remain with them in their doubt is not seeking to affirm their faith. To remain with them in their fear is refusing to be anxious, not striving to remove fear. To remain with them in their sadness is not insisting on wiping away their tears. To remain with them in their denial is to allow them the room to deny their deepest fear. Spiritual care does not seek to fix, but respects the sacredness of life in all its manifestations.

A colleague who has served as a chaplain for over twenty years tells me that, for him, chaplaincy is the art of just being there for patients, going with them where they wish to go. But, he states firmly, it is a difficult journey. When he first started his ministry, he was filled with theories and the need to fix, change, improve, and convert. I asked him why he changed. His reply was simple. He explained that one initially tries changing life to fit one's ideas. Then one learns that the reverse is true. We can't teach life. We can only learn from life.

The Importance of Being There

From a developmental perspective, change or transformation comes from within. Any external attempt to alter or improve remains superficial and temporary. Spiritual development is an individual journey. Like a wound that heals itself, the soul has its natural healing mechanisms. Given the right environment, it will naturally gravitate toward the healing process. Like Jung's internal archetype that guides the self toward wholeness, the soul moves toward healing. The calling of the caregiver is not to force the transition but to offer an environment that nurtures the soul. Henri Nouwen calls this environment "home." "Home is that place or space where we do not have to be afraid but can let go of our defenses and be free, free from worries, free from tensions, free from pressures."[6] Homelessness, according to Nouwen, is the inability to remain right where we are. It is a quest for a self that is not, a wish for something to be different. It is always in the future: "The tragedy is that we are so possessed by fear that we do not trust our innermost self as an intimate place but anxiously wander around hoping to find it where we are not. We try to find that intimate place in knowledge, competence, notoriety, success, friends, sensations, pleasure, dreams, or artificially induced states of consciousness. Thus we become strangers to ourselves."[7]

In a clinical context, homelessness can occur when we do not permit patients to scream, doubt, fear, cry, or be angry. When the natural expression of their affect is being monitored, it conveys the message that this affect and these thoughts and feelings are not acceptable. And when the reality of their affect is denied, the individual becomes homeless. Nouwen further points out that by offering a home that accommodates an individual fully, growth takes place. Within this home, one moves toward fecundity and fruitfulness. "Fruits . . . ask only for the rich soil, water, air, and sunlight of a caring environment in order to flourish."[8] Citing the example of Jesus, he writes, "Jesus cared deeply for the people he met. He did not control or dominate them, but through his words and actions offered them an opportunity to search for new directions."[9]

Space is the metaphor used by Ann Ulanov, professor of psychiatry and religion at Union Theological Seminary, to describe this therapeutic environment. Space is a place in between, a sacred place. With this space available, transition is possible. Without it, one may remain caught, arrested developmentally. This space, according to Ulanov, is the place between subjectivity and objectivity, feelings and facts, black and white, is and ought. In this in-between place, one is granted the liberty to just be without any coercion or persuasion to behave or feel one way or the other. It frees one to feel the depth of one's being without any form of judgment. Ulanov explains:

The psyche presses for its fulfillment. But this means including all our inferior parts, the undeveloped young parts. The stories in the New Testament, where God goes out into the highways and byways and brings in beggars, tax collectors, and whores to the dinner party, refer to us as individuals and to our existence in community. God brings the lowliest citizen to the highest place at the table. The parts of us and of our communities that grieve like widows, the parts of us we neglect like orphans—these, when included, bring wholeness. Whatever we run from will turn up in our subjective-object God-images. Whatever we fear will direct us to the place where God will find us. Whatever we skipped over and missed in psychological development we must go back and look for, for there God awaits us.[10]

It is through this space, affirms Ulanov, that we can meet God. "Only by attention to the space between our subjective-object God-images and the objective-object God-images of tradition can we discover the objective-subject God who awaits there, in that space, to meet us."[11]

When caregivers remain in the presence of the multiple ranges of feelings, reactions, and thoughts patients may be going through, they offer a sacred space, a home for souls in anguish. Through this space, transition is possible. Within this home, transformation becomes a possibility.

I was asked to see a client in a parenting program whose presenting problem, as indicated on the intake form, was childrearing. For four months of weekly sessions, she did not mention her children or indicate any desire to resolve problems related to parenting. For four months, she talked about her divorce, dating experiences, love life, and different guys she went out with, seeking my advice on who would be appropriate for her. I listened. With great curiosity as to why the conversation did not move in the direction indicated on the intake form, I was tempted to ask. Resisting the temptation, I kept listening. In the fifth month of our sessions, she no longer raised issues regarding her love life. She talked about her children and the problems they were facing, and our therapeutic relationship continued this way. Looking back, I now realize she needed space to be in touch with her deepest longings and pain. Only then was she able to make the necessary transition. Without that space, she would have remained arrested developmentally.

In D. W. Winnicott's paradigm, this client was given space to play, and through "play," health was restored. "It is play that is the universal, and that belongs to health: playing facilitates growth and therefore health; playing leads into group relationships; and playing can be a form of communication in psychotherapy."[12] However, in my personal reflections, I feel that the importance of space also extends into the realm of community.

Community and "Being There"

Community can play a significant role in the care of the soul or become the cause of anguish, thus perpetuating pathologies. In *Madness and Civilization*, Foucault helps us understand that it is not madness that leads to alienation but alienation that leads to madness. Here lies the significance of community.

In December 2003, I visited Thailand, intending to learn how Thai people who lack access to mental health facilities and psychological skills cope with trauma. I headed north and interviewed ten HIV-positive women from two northern provinces and four subdistricts. The outcome was not what I expected. When asked what helped them most, all ten responded with the same answer: support and acceptance from friends and family. A little girl told her mom that she would be there for her no matter how bad things might get. Many expected rejection from their families but were surprised to receive only support and encouragement. One woman was deeply depressed because she feared rejection by her community. But instead of rejection, her pastor and church members came to visit and pray for her. This brought great relief to her spirit.

Since support and acceptance from the community play a significant role in the healing process, the community needs to be aware of its power to include or alienate. This power emerges from the way the community defines the norm. By drawing a line, we include some and exclude others. The more criteria we have, the smaller our drawn circle, leaving a greater number of people on the outside, rejected and alienated. Each community needs to come to realize that norms are not the most essential. They change from place to place, culture to culture, denomination to denomination, and religion to religion. Therefore, norms need to be viewed as guidelines. Instead of drawing solid lines, we need to draw dotted ones. In a setting where believers are not permitted to be angry at God or to express doubt, the community can cause great harm by not providing a sacred space for traumatized individuals to fully experience the entire range of their emotions. By not being there to offer a home for anguished souls, the community can become a force that retards the spiritual growth of individuals. Instead of promoting transition, a community can actually cause a person to go into spiritual regression.

Spiritual Care: Methods

From this perspective, spiritual care is the art of creating sacred space for individuals who are attempting to make sense of their reality. Caregivers need to be conscious of the fact that whenever they are in the presence of someone who is in pain, who has been informed that he or she has limited time left, and just learned that he or she has symptoms that may not go away, reality lies beyond appearances. The space the individual occupies may be filled with feelings, thoughts, fears, anxieties, anger, doubts, obsessions, questions, and a host of other related issues. Introjection may prohibit him or her from experiencing or exploring certain thoughts or emotions. His or her theology may not permit doubt or questioning God. Socialization may make it impossible for the person to express anger. Cultural norms may dictate that he or she needs to appear strong. His or her space may already be occupied by internal scripts, limiting the availability of much-needed space in which to process matters and move on. Awareness of what takes place within the space beyond appearances is an important step.

One of the most important gifts a caregiver can bring is an empty self without words or actions. Simple presence can communicate something much more beneficial than careful selection of words or well-strategized deeds. People can normally tell whether a caregiver is coming in with or without an agenda. When we come with an empty self, patients can breathe better in the safe environment of the sacred space we are offering them. James Dittes gives this description:

> The counselor is content to be a witness, not a player. The counselor is intensely present to the counselee, but as a witness. The counselor does not crave or design to have an impact, to make a difference, or to leave his or her mark on the counselee's life. Nor does the counselor aspire to find satisfaction, community, or accomplishment. Aspirations that may be perfectly appropriate in everyday conversations—to be curious, to assuage pain, to solve problems, to master perplexities, to understand and know and explain why things are the way they are, to be loved and admired and understood—are put on hold.[13]

To be empty is to step in with no expectations of one's performance as a caregiver. Caregiving is not about determining how a session should go, how a patient should react, or having a preconceived idea of a positive or negative response. The empty self does not seek to gain anything for itself, not even the knowledge of helping to improve the situation. The empty self remains empty, thus allowing natural processes to take place within the patient.

Creating space is an art for which certain skills may be helpful. Ordinarily, when we talk about being there for others, we think of offering words of comfort. An elderly lady who grieved the death of her husband often mentioned the guilt she was experiencing to her family members. In attempting to be there for her, their response was, "You do not have to feel guilty. You did your best. You did not do anything wrong." It was a loving attempt at consolation, but it took away the space she needed for grieving and the guilt she needed to feel and process. When I met her, she had stopped talking about her guilt to her family members altogether. But that guilt had remained strong, creating various negative emotions. What she needed was space in which to explore her sense of guilt, express her feelings about it, and come to terms with it. A more helpful approach was to explore her sense of guilt with her, letting her talk about what she was feeling and thinking.

This is also true with experiences of denial, anger, doubt, and fear. Often we are acculturated to break down denial, not realizing that it plays an important role in sustaining a person's psyche. When my dad knew he was dying, he talked to us about his funeral and preparations for it only twice. Most of the time he talked about his plans for the future, a future he knew would never take place. For a while I was puzzled by his behavior, until I realized that each of us can take only so much pain. Once the pain is contained, one is more able to face reality. It is also interesting to note that the psyche's ability to cope with pain is fluid. A person may be more able to cope on one day than another. Denial helps protect and sustain until the individual is ready to face troubling issues. Elizabeth Kubler-Ross writes, "Denial functions as a buffer after unexpected shocking news, allows the patient to collect himself and, with time, mobilize other, less radical defenses,"[14] because "denial is usually a temporary defense and will soon be replaced by partial acceptance."[15] In the presence of denial, "being there" for patients suggests a willingness to remain with them even in their denial. If they want to talk about their future plans, talk about their future plans. If they want to fantasize about recovery, fantasize with them. Reflecting on the case of Mrs. K. who was caught in a stage of deep denial, Kubler-Ross concludes:

Looking back at this long and meaningful relationship, I am sure that it was possible only because she sensed that we respected her wish to deny her illness as long as possible. We never became judgmental no matter how much of a management problem she presented. . . . In the long run it is the persistent nurturing role of the therapist who has dealt with his or her own death complex sufficiently that helps the patient overcome the anxiety and fear of his impending death.[16]

The same attitude can be applied to anger, doubt, and fear. Denying a person's anger does not make it go away. Accommodating by not being reactive or taking it personally helps individuals process their anger. When people are given a proper channel for their anger, it becomes manageable. When anger is viewed as inappropriate and totally negative, it has no place to go except to regress. Similarly, doubt has to be explored, and fear experienced. Doubt does not go away with rational explanation. Existential doubt needs to be explored existentially, because this type of doubt emerges from being and is not a theoretical concern. Therefore, answers have to be felt and experienced.

Speaking of existential doubt and fear reminds me of a story told by Allison J. Nichols about her dying friend who had cancer of the lung, kidney, and liver. She appeared stoic and prayed frequently during her illness. One day she informed Allison of a dream she had had. She was carrying a huge giftbox up to a church located on a hilltop. As she was climbing, she kept falling back. But she persisted. Finally, she reached the top and, as she made her way into the church, the box kept knocking other parishioners on their heads. An elderly man with a white beard came over and asked her to lay the box down at the altar. She refused, grabbed the box, and left the church. After relating this dream, she asked Allison about the meaning of it. In return, Allison asked what was inside the box. Together they both imagined themselves untying the big red bow.

With tears streaming down her fragile face, she looked into the box and told me that it was filled with garbage. Spontaneously, she cried out to God, "What have I done to deserve this? Where are you? I can't stand this anymore. I hate you!"

My friend did not need me to interpret her dream. She understood, at the deepest level, that the garbage symbolized all the negative feelings that she was denying God. She knew too that the wise man in her dream was urging her to leave the box on the altar as a gift to God.

The next morning my dying friend smiled as I entered her room. She couldn't wait to tell me what had happened during the night. With her mouth so dry and cracked that she could hardly speak, she told me that she had looked across the room at the wall facing her bed and saw a beautiful young man with long blonde hair. He was standing in a field of wildflowers—beckoning to her.[17]

Her cry was an affirmation of faith and respect for the God big enough to accommodate her fears, doubts, and anger. "Her prayer showed enough trust in God's love to express her rage at God for the horrors that she simply did not understand."[18]

During my ten years of teaching spiritual care to health-care students at Loma Linda University, the topic of prayer has led to much discussion and debate from a variety of perspectives. The conversation often centers on the issue of miracles and intervention. As I grapple with the concept of prayer in the clinical context, I have come to a greater appreciation of the message conveyed in Allison's story. I have learned that the more concrete our description of the full depth of what we are going through, the more healing takes place. In the context of spiritual care, prayer needs to take us to the depths of our struggle so that we actually feel our spirituality and the texture of our soul. For the caregiver to offer prayer is to show patients that God is indeed willing to provide a sacred space for them to experience fully their entire being. Prayer invites them to open themselves fully to God in every dimension of their struggle; it conveys to them that in God's presence they can cry, weep, fear, doubt, scream, shout, and feel, just feel. The place of prayer is the gift of removing all the oughts and shoulds from the equation so one can just be. The way we pray can have an important role in facilitating this process. In the poetic wisdom of Jewel Kilcher,

> Prayer is the greatest
> Swiftest
> Ship my heart could sail upon.[19]

Conclusion

The invitation to provide spiritual care is a call to be with individuals who are going through trauma and attempting to make sense of their new reality. We offer them a safe space that nurtures their soul while they struggle with the many aspects of their experience. Here we do not attempt to fix, cure, or resolve their wounds. Neither do we tell them not to feel guilty or be afraid, not to doubt but to have faith, not to get angry but to be calm. Here we stay with them as they make this difficult journey into the depths of their being. This is where care of the soul takes place in the ministry of healing. The offering of sacred space as individuals struggle with sickness can bring healing to souls that yearn for the quality of depth in the midst of suffering itself.

Appendixes

Endnotes

Bibliography

Index

Definition of Terms

Alchemy   The medieval chemical philosophy that seeks transformation of base metals into gold. In psychological terms, Jung sees alchemy as the path whereby human spirits, through a painful process, are transformed from ignorance to enlightenment.

Bhagavad Gita   Sacred book in the Hindu tradition. It forms a part of the Mahabharata and contains the story of Krishna (the incarnation of Lord Vishnu) giving advice to Arjuna on the meaning of life while on the battlefield.

Coniunctio   In the language of alchemy, coniunctio refers to the unity of elements with opposite qualities, such as man and woman, light and darkness, black and white.

Dharma   Dharma, in Buddhism, refers to the teaching of the Buddha regarding the nature of reality and how one ought to live in accord with it.

Infallible   Unable to fail, not erroneous, incapable of being wrong or mistaken.

Kali   The goddess of destruction, a consort of Lord Shiva. To her worshippers, she destroys ignorance, greed, and materialism while supporting those who pursue true understanding.

Kundalini   The literal meaning of kundalini is "coiling," and it implies the untapped energy or potential within each one of us. It also describes the vital and sexual energy that resides within our unconscious self.

Labyrinth   The unicursal labyrinth can be dated back many thousands of years and contains religious meaning. It has only one entrance leading to the center and one exit point. There are normally three forms of labyrinth: the seven, eleven, and twelve circuits. There is a 180- degree angle for every turn in each circuit (implying the need to shift consciousness). It is believed that walking the labyrinth helps to balance and add depth to one's soul.

Lingum   The phallus symbol, which represents the creative power of primal energy of Lord Shiva.

Logos   The word logos in Greek is literally translated as "the word." The term is used by Panikkar to refer to the power of reasoning.

Making merits   The performing good deeds to compensate for wrongs done in order to acquire a greater possibility of entering into a better place in another life.

Mandala   In Sanskrit, mandala means "circle." It is a symbol of the universe and its cosmic forces. In Jungian psychology, mandala represents wholeness. Jung believed that mandala is archetypal. It forms a part of our psyche, our being. It is a symbol that guides us toward wholeness.

Ontology   Philosophical exploration of the nature of being and human existence.

Pica   A form of eating disorder commonly found among children with developmental issues. Individuals with pica will ingest non-nutritional substances such as dirt, clay, hair, stones, etc.

Praxis   Application of one's theoretical knowledge.

Tao   It is literally translated as "the Way." In Taoism, it refers to that which contains everything and excludes nothing. It is all embracing. It is what it is. And in being what it is, it guides us to seek to align ourselves with nature.

Yin and Yang   Yin and yang symbolize the two opposing forces that co-exist. Yin refers to that which is dark, soft, passive, and feminine; yang, to light, energy, and the masculine. The yin and yang concept points to the structure of the universe that contains both elements and the need for us to learn to maintain the tension between them as we go through life.

Yoni   In Sanskrit, means "holder." Yoni is the female sexual organ that represents the goddess Sakti, the consort of Lord Shiva. This symbol is often seen in relation to lingum (symbolizing the coexistence of two opposite elements).

Ontology and Spirituality | Raimundo Panikkar,
Paul Tillich, and Carl Jung

Raimundo Panikkar: The Function and Goals of Myth

Function

In attempting to explain Panikkar's interpretation of the function of myth, I will look at his explanation of myth and ideology, myth and morality, and the myth of *Prajapati*.[1]

In his discussion of myth and ideology, Panikkar summarizes the role of myth:

You can tolerate in a positive and total way only what you accept. Now you can accept only what you either understand with the *logos* or embrace in myth. In the first case, i.e., if and insofar as you understand, there is no need to tolerate. On the other hand, positive tolerance has to do with what you accept fully without understanding it. Here is the place and the role of myth. Communion in the same myth is what makes tolerance possible.[2]

This statement shows that myth makes tolerance possible because myth accepts fully without having the desire to fully understand. Logos (logic) cannot remain the sole ground for tolerance, since rationality cannot tolerate contradiction and polarity. To believe that truth is completely objective is to lack the ability to fully accept that which cannot be assimilated into logic. A similar argument is reflected in Panikkar's explication of morality. "The 'primitive' follows his myth without question. The day he begins to ask why, he attains knowledge of good and evil and immediately becomes aware of the unreasonable, irrational character of myth."[3] Rationality disintegrates morality. The moment we seek a rational basis for morality, we discover that there is no ground to stand on. It is "myth" that sustains morality and not rationality.[4] Hence, myth makes morality possible.

In the section on the myth of *Prajapati,* the myth of pain implies, "We suffer and we find in this suffering a value that transcends anything that a physical and psychic causality might propose."[5] This myth is rooted in the nature of our beings. The problem is when we attempt to explain it; we lose sight of the purifying process and redemptive function of pain. If God is the Ultimate, then everything must come from God. If sin originates in God, we are powerless to fight against sin. Hence, there is no explanation for the problem of pain. But in "myth," God remains the Ultimate Reality and yet not the originator of sin. This redemptive function of pain is rooted not in our rationality but in our mythology, as illustrated in the myth of *Prajapati.*

The myth of *Prajapati* helps us see that sin does not originate in God. The act of creation is God's annihilation of God into nothing. The result of this falling into nothing is humanity or, in the words of Panikkar, "Man who finds himself as if floating between a nothing that 'was' and a God who 'will be.'"[6] In the act of giving birth, there occurred an originating fault. This fault is provisional. It is not sin. It becomes "sin" only when we take this provisional state to be definite. God is on the way to becoming God through humanity. It is through this process that we come to understand pain and the myth of pain.

Myth that is derived from the inherent structure of being makes tolerance of others possible, sustains morality, upholds the belief in a great and supreme God as the Creator of all, and yet leaves room for an explanation of pain. This possibility takes place because myth provides direct access to reality without having to go through reason. From these three examples of myth, we can clearly see that the function of myth as a transcendental element, located in our ontological structure, is to direct life to its maximum functionality.

Goal

Panikkar's elucidation of the word "wisdom" offers an insight into his understanding of the role of myth:

The oft-decried homelessness of the modern person results from the fact that scientific cosmology is not able to offer the person a human dwelling place. The scientific world is no dwelling place. The person is lost in the quantitative desert of an "expanding" universe and the chain of millions of years reaching back to our animal ancestors. The person is homeless because the scientific worldview has lost the human dimension, and even more so because this worldview's dwelling place has not been erected by wisdom but by an extrapolating calculation.[7]

Myth, like wisdom, is not based on the scientific worldview. Myth emerges naturally from the heart and seeks to direct life while aiming to bring about an understanding of spirituality that correlates with each individual's ontic reality. The spiritual goal of human beings is explained in the third mytheme[8] in "The Myth of the Human Condition." Part of the human being consists of desire, which is "the manifestation of each being's deepest dynamism."[9] This desire is transcendental, since it is "neither caprice nor the consequence of a reasoning intellect, but the result of an integral situation."[10] This transcendental desire represents the longing for what will engage one's entire being and can best be described as the "ontological tendency of every being"[11] that "expresses the ontological structure of human existence."[12]

This transcendental desire refers to the desire to be. The desire to be here refers to the desire for authenticity of life in contrast to inauthentic life. Inauthentic life is a life that has been conditioned by the fear of death and the attachment to life. It is, as Tillich suggests, the result of the anxiety of nonbeing, which threatens the ontic (in terms of death) and spiritual (in terms of meaninglessness) self-affirmation of human beings.[13] Humanity has been conditioned by fear, pain, anxiety, death, and attachment. It is in submitting oneself to these conditions that humanity has ceased to be in an authentic way. It is in this light that we come to an understanding of the goal of myth, which "describes the human condition in order to present the deconditioning of Man as its quintessential message."[14] Myth helps us understand our condition and at the same time points us to the desire deep within each of us. "In the depths of this ontological desire true human freedom dwells."[15] The desired freedom is the freedom from the conditions of life that inauthenticates life itself. Only through freedom can human beings truly be. Only through freedom does authenticity become a possibility. The achievement of this freedom is reflected in the myth of Sunahsepa[16] and his willingness to sacrifice his life. It is also found in the teachings of Jesus when he says: "For whoever wants to save his life will lose it, but whoever loses his life for me and for the gospel will save it" (Mark 8:35). My reflection on Panikkar's concept of freedom has led me to the understanding that being is finite. Time is temporal. Space is limited. Pain and suffering remind us of our nonbeing and finiteness. To accept nonbeing is to encounter Being. To Panikkar, only through our willingness to give our lives can we regain authenticity of self. Sunahsepa achieved life because he was willing to sacrifice his life. This myth reveals to us that the "price of this true freedom is our own life."[17] Panikkar confirms the most powerful symbol of Christianity when he suggests that true spirituality is the achievement of the freedom to be that takes place when one is willing to lay down one's life.[18] True spirituality is contained in the symbol of the cross.

Paul Tillich and the Structure of Being

Human Transition from Essence to Existence

To Tillich, this deep yearning for meaning is rooted in the fact that human beings are not where they ought to be. They are not what they ought to be because of sin. Tillich does not think of sin in a traditional sense. Sin is rooted in the structure of being. We are created to be free. Freedom implies the power to contradict oneself and one's essential nature, so freedom creates the possibility of transition from essence to existence. Essence here means potentiality and the possibility of actualization of human potential. Through the awareness of freedom and, at the same time, the possibility of death and suffering, the self seeks to actualize itself through decision making. In this process, the self moves from an essential state to an estranged state of being because there will always be biological, sociological, and psychological forces affecting an individual's decision. This Tillich refers to as "the fall." This fall is not only an event that took place in the past; it is continually happening in every existential decision.

Human Existential Self-Destruction and Despair

To Tillich, the basic expression of human existential state of unbelief,[19] hubris,[20] and concupiscence[21] contradicts human essential being and drives the polar elements of this being into conflict with each other. Consequently, the estranged state contains within itself the structures of destruction, which aims at chaos. The state of estrangement leads to a sense of despair, because under this condition, the polar opposites turn demonic and destructive.

Christ

Human beings in the state of existential estrangement cannot restore themselves and regain their essential state of being. This can only be accomplished through revelation which takes place through the New Being. This New Being is reflected in Christ in that although he took on all the infirmities of human finitude, he conquered them through courage to be in the face of nonbeing. He remained united with God under all conditions and did not give in to faithlessness, hubris, and concupiscence.

Christ accepted the conditions of his existence (nonbeing and finitude), but overcame them. Hence, he became the power of New Being. When one is grasped by the power of the New Being, three things take place:

1. Regeneration is objectively the New Being itself, and subjectively, the individual's rebirth or transformation through participation in the power of the new reality as it is made manifest in Christ. Through Christ, one has faith instead of unbelief, surrender instead of hubris, and love instead of concupiscence.

2. Justification. Objectively, this is the eternal act of God by which he accepts individuals as not being estranged, as opposed to those who are indeed estranged from him by guilt. It is the act by which God takes them into unity with himself as manifested in the New Being. Subjectively, this refers to human beings accepting that they are accepted.

3. Sanctification. Sanctification is the process through which salvation actually works itself out in history. It is the process whereby the power of the New Being transforms personality and community, inside and outside the church.

Through Christ, as the symbol of New Being, human beings now accept their finitude and the negativities inherent in it without rebellion. As a result, hope, instead of despair, becomes their final attitude.

Carl Jung and the Religious Function of the Psyche

To Jung, the human psyche contains a religious function essential for growth and development. The psyche is structured in polarities. In order to achieve wholeness, the ego must recognize and reconcile these polarities. The process of reconciliation occurs through conscious participation in symbols that emerge from the unconscious and bring together two opposing poles in a third form. This new symbol brings consciousness to a deeper level by being in touch with the rest of the psyche, enhancing relationships with others and the self. The religious function, therefore, is the capacity of the psyche to produce symbols that have this reconciling effect and stirring presence.[22]

The religious function of the psyche can be described as a drive toward relations between the personal self to the transpersonal source of the meaning and power of being. If this drive does not find fulfillment, it will express itself through symptoms of neurosis.

Religious Function of the Psyche

According to Jung, the religious function expresses itself in clear and distinct ways. First, it expresses itself through a direct personal experience of the numinous. The numinous imposes itself on the individual, often in a dream, drawing, vision, or event. One feels its impact through images and affects rather than through concepts. The experience of the numinous is non-rational. The individual feels that the mysterious symbolism is greater than him- or herself, and yielding to the power of this symbol brings peace of mind. Second, the religious function expresses itself in translating the original numinous experience into dogmas and creeds. The symbols of dogma express an intensely lived psychic reality.

Transcendent Function of the Psyche

The religious function is the capacity of the psyche to produce symbols that point a person toward wholeness. This process is best understood in Jung's description of the "transcendent function." Transcendent function refers to the tendencies of the unconscious mind to guide, through symbolism, to the process of inviduation. The task of the therapist is to bring consciousness and unconsciousness together to arrive at a new attitude.

The Unconscious and Religion

Jung's description of the transcendent function is similar to his understanding of the religious function of the psyche. At this point, I would like to place this understanding of the transcendent function in the context of Jung's understanding of religion. To Jung, religion is a necessary fact of human experience. Religion is derived from *religare*, which means "to bind back" or "to bind strongly." According to Ann and Barry Ulanov, religion binds us "to the immediate, primordial experience of the numinous that seizes and controls the human subject. One may feel fear, awe, love, and adoration toward the numinous, but one accepts the necessity of its effect on day-to-day living."[23]

Jung believes that religion provides two kinds of balance protection. It safeguards human sanity through of tradition and dogma; and keeps records of experiences of the divine. Secondly, it provides the individual with a frame of reference which transcends the mass-mindedness of modern society, protecting the individual from submersion in the mass.[24]

Jung also recognizes that religion assists in a transition from protection to a more objective understanding of God. "God may at first contain projections of our own wishes and operate as pseudo-satisfaction for our own fantasies. But reality teaches us to place God outside our own control just as we learn to do with any other object. This means that we, as subjects, notice that God, the object, has survived destruction as a mere extension of our projections."[25] Here we come to acknowledge God's existence apart from our protection.

Religion also helps us deal with our projection of evil. When we project evil we may think that our life is filled with happiness that has no pain or misery. But when we withdraw our projection, we see the "otherness" of God and realize the mysterious nature of evil. We no longer see evil as a problem to be solved, and realize that God cannot be identified with human concepts of goodness.[26]

Religious Function and the Healthy Human Psyche

The religious function, as has been described above, plays an important role in restoring health to the human psyche. Its importance to the human psyche is reflected, first, in positive projection. The religious function seems to be pointing to the place of paradox. This paradox is not something to be solved, but is something to be contained, and its containment is what provides healing for the human psyche. "We do not have to reduce ourselves to live at the conceptual level alone, which is the level that must resolve all paradox, or compulsively turn mysteries into problems that can be explained away."[27] Religion allows our contact with otherness to evolve slowly. It encourages toleration of non-directed thinking. It allows for the working of the unconscious. It helps us to be in touch with the "otherness" of the numinous. Second, the religious function points to new possibilities for life. With the acceptance of the two levels of psychic functioning, the conscious and the unconscious, new possibilities for spiritual development are opened to us. Through the religious function of the psyche, one learns to differentiate and separate the unconscious and conscious elements. One differentiates not in order to get rid of one or endorse the other: both belong to the human psyche. In the process of differentiation, we no longer believe that a desire is conquered simply because it has become unconscious. Rather, we accept the fact that we have desires, needs, and wishes with all their accompanying erotic imagery, driving passions, and compelling action. In this recognition, we are no longer slaves to them. We are free from their power over us.[28]

Diagnosis of Søren Kierkegaard

In my attempt at diagnosing Søren Kierkegaard (*DSM* is utilized merely as a guide for reflection and not as a final definitive tool for arriving at the truth about the person), I experienced an irresistible urge to define my limitations. A Kierkegaard scholar once mentioned that understanding Kierkegaard is the work of a century. This appendix does not represent a century of study. Second, "Kierkegaard is difficult to read, very difficult indeed. That was his intention, and he got his way."[1] Finally, if Fenger's studies of the original documents were correct when he said "of course, Kierkegaard had the right to suppress, rewrite, misrepresent, distort, erase, destroy, and lead astray, and to arrange the interpretation of his life and his works,"[2] no diagnosis is possible without clearly defined limitations. My diagnosis is based primarily on two biographies, Walter Lowrie's *A Short Life of Kierkegaard* and Josiah Thompson's *Kierkegaard*.

Important Variables in the Life of Søren Kierkegaard

Mental Health: Constant complaints of melancholy, derealization, feelings of sadness, emptiness, fear of losing control, fear of going crazy, history of mental illness (brother and nieces) and constant fear and worries related to light, temperature, sound, and fire.[3]

Physical Health: Tuberculosis (staphylococcus infection), indigestion, and physical appearance.

Stressful Events: Upbringing, deaths of five of his siblings, deaths of his parents, breaking his engagement, attack by the *Corsair*, and his "earthquake experience."

The following list includes dates and important events in Kierkegaard's life:

Date	Event
May 5, 1813	SK was born.
1819	Søren Michael died at age 12 (bumping his head).
1822	Maren Kirsten died of cramps at age 24.
October 30, 1830	Entered University of Copenhagen.
September 10, 1832	Nicoline Christine died giving birth.
Sept. 21, 1833	Niels Andreas died in his 25th year.
April 15, 1834	Started his journals.
July 31, 1834	His mother died.
December 29, 1834	Petrea Severine died at 33 giving birth to a son.
May 1835	The "great earthquake."
May 1837	Met Regina.
May 1838	Entered in his journal: "indescribable joy."
August 9, 1838	His father died.
July–August 1840	Journeyed to Jutland.
September 10, 1840	Engaged to Regina.
October 11, 1841	Broke his engagement
July 1843	Learned of Regina's engagement
January 1845	Corsair attacks.
November 1847	Regina married F. Schlegel.
April 1848	Discovered forgiveness
June 1852	Content with being different.
November 4, 1855	SK died.

Reading Kierkegaard's biographies led me to the conclusion that perhaps he was suffering from a mood disorder, perhaps dysthymic disorder with an early onset. He most likely experienced two major depressive episodes[4] (discovering his father's curse and sexuality, and during the *Corsair* affair) and had an obsessive-compulsive personality.

Differential Diagnosis

1. Was the mood disorder a part of him or did it start with the "earthquake experience"? Lowrie and psychiatrist Hjalmar Helweg believe that he experienced a normal childhood and that depression set in during his "earthquake experience."[5] In my personal opinion, Kierkegaard experienced the deaths of five of his siblings and the death of his mother before the earthquake experience. And he exhibited some sort of mood disorder prior to the earthquake experience. Was this experience the final straw in his struggle with the many deaths in his family, the deaths that ostensibly came as a punishment from God? This is a possibility. I am inclined to think that the earthquake experience is related to his first major depressive episode.

2. Were his symptoms the result of acute stress disorder, a panic disorder, or a dissociative disorder? Variables I have tried to sort out are derealization, a sense of detachment, fear of losing control, fear of going crazy, fear of dying, worries, etc. What needs to be determined is whether these symptoms of anxiety were caused by external events, or if he inherited an anxiety-prone personality.

The deaths of most of his family members (five of his six siblings and both of his parents) were traumatic experiences. On top of this, he was brought up with an outlook that was dark, gloomy, and extremely pessimistic; he was brought up "crazily," as he himself described it. These choices are very tempting options—namely, acute stress disorder, panic disorder, and depersonalization disorder—since all three provide possible explanations for his frequent complaints of fear of losing control, fear of going crazy, derealization, fear of death, or any threat to life. I am more inclined toward panic disorder for the following reasons:

a. He did not meet criteria G for acute stress disorder.[6]

b. Although he meets all criteria stated under 300.6 (depersonalization disorder) with the exception of criteria D, the derealization he was experiencing was an ongoing thing throughout his entire life instead of occurring immediately after a traumatic life-threatening experience.

c. The cause of depersonalization disorder is often associated with a life-threatening experience, which Kierkegaard did experience, but depersonalization is also a part of panic disorder. Panic disorder can better account for his fear of dying, light, fire, noise and uneven temperature.[7] Further, he had a family history of insanity. His brother, the bishop, became dysfunctional and had to quit his work for a period of time. His nephews had many insanity attacks, and one of them committed suicide.

My inclination toward panic disorder is not fully justified because, according to his journals and biographies, there is no mention of panic attacks that developed abruptly. Nevertheless, he exhibited at least four of the symptoms.

Panic Attack

a. Sweating: Fenger makes reference to Kierkegaard's "nocturnal perspiration."[8]

b. Derealization: Thompson states: "His problem . . . is how to stop that leak, how to prevent consciousness from 'sneaking out of the world.'"[9]

c. Fear of losing control or going crazy: On May 8, 1837, he wrote, "I thank thee, O Lord, that when thou over lookest me thou did not let me go mad at once,—I have never been so afraid of it." And on May 17, 1843, he observed: "Had I had faith I should have remained with Regina. Thanks and praise be to God, I now see that. I was near to losing my mind in those days."[10]

d. Fear of dying: On October 13, 1853, he wrote in his journal: "I thought I should die very young." And on a scrap paper, upon reflecting on his father's sin, he wrote: "A sort of presentiment commonly precedes everything that is to happen; but just as this may have a deterrent effect, so also it may have a tempting effect, for the fact that it awakens in a person the thought that he is predestined, as it were, he sees himself carried on through a chain of consequences, but consequences over which he has no control." The implication of these statements is clear when we realize that his father perceived the deaths in the family as God's punishment. And it was in this context that Kierkegaard saw himself as "the object of the fury of the angry gods."[11]

Dysthymic Disorder: 300.4[12]

1. Being depressed for at least two years: In *Point of View for My Work as an Author*, he writes: "It's really awful when a man's consciousness has borne such a weight from childhood that neither the soul's elasticity nor its freedom can throw it off. . . . He who has borne such a weight from childhood on is like a child who has been taken from its mother with forceps and who always bears a physical trace of the mother's pain."[13]

2. Two or more related symptoms

a. Insomnia: This is indicated by Fenger in *Kierkegaard: Myths and Their Origin*, page 66.

b. Low self-esteem: In describing Kierkegaard, Regina writes: "He was tortured by the thought that he had not been good enough to his father, whom he loved enormously."[14] Besides, he was constantly troubled by his physical appearance. He asked his cousin, Christian Kierkegaard, to draw two idealized portraits of himself.

c. Poor concentration or experiencing difficulty in the decision making process: This was clearly reflected in his relationship with Regina. He had a difficult time, moving back and forth between wanting to get married and yet wondering if marriage would be the best thing for both of them.

d. Hopelessness: "How terrible tedium is . . . I lie stretched out inactive; the only thing I see is emptiness. The only thing I feed on is emptiness. I do not even suffer pain."[15]

3. Experiencing symptoms as stated in the above criteria for more than two months during the period of disturbance: There seems to be no indication that he had been with or without these symptoms for more than two months. Feelings of joy and peace were described only a few times in his entire life.

4. No major depressive episode during the first two years: Even as a child, Kierkegaard complained of his melancholy: "My life began without any immediate experience, with a terrible melancholy in earliest childhood deranged in its deepest foundations." The following year, he wrote, "I never knew the joy of being a child."[16]

5. The symptoms caused clinically significant distress in social, occupational, and other areas of his life. In describing his melancholy, he writes, "I had my thorn in the flesh, and therefore did not marry and could not take on an official position."[17]

Major Depressive Episode (after his "earthquake experience")

1. Depressed mood most of the day: Thomson described Kierkegaard during this period: "Instead of becoming rich and full, however, his interior life became poor and empty. At this time he began speaking of his consciousness as 'far too roomy' . . . he remarked 'My head is as dead and empty as a theater after the performance is over.'"[18]

a. Lack of interest or pleasure: "without any expectation of leading a happy earthly life, without hope of a happy and comfortable future."[19]

b. Insomnia: Kierkegaard's insomnia is recorded in Fenger's *Kierkegaard: Myths and Their Origin*, page 66.

c. Fatigue or loss of energy: "I don't feel like doing anything; I don't feel like walking—it tires me out; I don't feel like lying down; for either I should lie down for a long time, or I should get up again right away, and I don't feel at all like doing that."[20]

d. Recurrent thoughts of death: "I've just returned from a party of which I was the life and soul; wit poured from my lips, everyone laughed and admired me—but I went away—and the dash should be as long as the earth's orbit . . . and I wanted to shoot myself."[21]

2. His symptoms did not meet criteria for a mixed episode.

3. The symptoms caused significant distress in his life: "At the present time I live like a chess piece of which the opponent says: that piece cannot be moved—as an idle onlooker, for my time is not yet come."[22]

4. The symptoms were not the result of substance abuse.

5. The symptoms were not the result of bereavement, i.e., loss of a loved one, and they persisted for longer than two months.

Obsessive-Compulsive Personality Disorder

Obsessive-compulsive personality disorder refers to a pattern of obsession with orderliness, cleanliness, perfection, and control, lacking in flexibility and openness. This pattern normally starts during early adulthood and presented itself in a variety of ways in Kierkegaard's life. He was:

1. Occupied with details: Discussing Kierkegaard's environment, Thompson writes: "[B]ack in Copenhagen not a detail was neglected to construct an environment perfectly suited to Kierkegaard's wishes."[23]

2. Excessively devoted to work: This is revealed in the quantity of the writing he produced during his short life in contrast to his social life.

3. Overconscientious and inflexible in matters relating to morality, ethics, or values: Lowrie describes Kierkegaard thus: "It is certain that he had a rare sense of shame, and possibly he was more distressed by the impure suggestions of sensuality than most men are."[24]

4. Rigidity and stubbornness: Kierkegaard's polemical characteristic was exhibited from his childhood days, when he was described as a "wild cat," and it stayed with him until the end.

Multiaxial Evaluation Report

Axis I: Clinical Disorders

296.3	Major depressive disorder, recurrent without full interepisode recovery, superimposed on dysthamic disorder
300.4	Dysthamic disorder with early onset
300.01	Panic disorder (suggested possibility)

Axis II: Personality Disorders

301.4	Obsessive-compulsive personality disorder

Axis III: General Medical Conditions

011.9	Tuberculosis
714.0	Arthritis, rheumatoid (?)

Axis IV: Psychosocial and Environmental Problems

Problem with primary support group: death of siblings and parents.
Problems related to the social environment: inadequate social support and difficulty with acculturation.
GAF = 50

Notes

Introduction

1. A popular beach located southeast of Bangkok, Thailand.

2. Leo Buscaglia. *Living, Loving and Learning* (New York: Fawcett Columbine, 1982), 91.

3. A study by Oleckno and Blacconiere assessing one thousand university students in Illinois found that religious students are healthier, with fewer injuries and less cigarette, alcohol, and drug use. They reported fewer illnesses and demonstrated greater conformity to rules. W. A. Oleckno and M. J. Blacconiere, "Relationship of Religiosity to Wellness and Other Health-Related Behaviors and Outcomes," *Psychological Reports* 68 (1991): 819–26. Another study of cancer patients shows that highly religious people tend to report more life satisfaction and happiness and indicate less pain in comparison to less religious patients. J. W. Yates, B. J. Chalmer, P. St. James et al., "Religion in Patients with Advanced Cancer," *Medical Pediatric Oncology* 9 (1981): 121–28. Sixteen studies have also found a correlation between worship attendance, religiosity, and low blood pressure. Harold G. Koenig, *Spirituality in Patient Care: Why, How, When, and What* (Philadelphia: Templeton Foundation Press, 2002), 11. A study by Oxman and colleagues investigating persons over the age of sixty with heart disease undergoing bypass surgery shows the overall mortality rate of 9 percent at six months. However, the rate drops to 5 percent among churchgoers and to 0 percent for those who are deeply religious. T. E. Oxman, D. H. Freeman, and E. D. Manheimer, "Lack of Social Participation or Religious Strength and Comfort as Risk Factors for Death after Cardiac Surgery in the Elderly," *Psychosomatic Medicine* 57 (1995): 5–15. For more studies on the relationship of religion, spirituality, and health, see the following: H. G. Koenig, "Religious Beliefs and Practices of Hospitalized Medically Ill Older Adults," *International Journal of Geriatric Psychiatry* 13 (1998): 213–24; H. G. Koenig, L. K. George, and B. L. Peterson, "Religiosity and Remission of Depression in Medically Ill Older Patients," *American Journal of Psychiatry* 155 (1998): 536–42; H. G. Koenig, "Use of Acute Hospital Services and Mortality Among Religious and Non-Religious Copers with Medical Illness," *Journal of Religious Gerontology* 9 (1995): 1–22; K. Pargament et al., "God Help Me (I): Religious Coping Efforts as Predictors of the Outcomes of Significant Negative Life Events, *American Journal of Community Psychology,* 18 (1990): 793–824; K. Pargament, H. G. Koenig, N. Tarakeshwar, and J. Hahn, "Religious Struggle as a Predictor of Mortality among Medically Ill Elderly Patients: A Two-Year Longitudinal Study," *Archives of Internal Medicine* 161 (2001): 881–85.

Chapter One

1. Cited by Douglas Dales, "Celtic and Anglo-Saxon Spirituality," in Gordon Mursell, ed., *The Story of Christian Spirituality: Two Thousand Years, From East to West* (Minneapolis: Fortress Press, 2002), 78.

2. Cited by Bradley Holt, "Spiritualities of the Twentieth Century," in Mursell, ed., *The Story of Christian Spirituality*, 319.

3. Cited by Sergei Hacked, "The Russian Spirit," in Mursell, ed., *The Story of Christian Spirituality*, 116.

4. A close friend of mine often finds this obligation depressing. Having to spend time with God is very different from wanting to spend time with God. There are those who like to spend time with God and there are those who do not. In regards to God, we almost have to like who this God is, or feel damnation if we do not express a sense of appreciation in some form. Further reflection seems to indicate that it is not just spending time with God that enriches one's spirituality. The reverse is often true in that it is *who* we spend time with and not how often or how much. But again, this is only one view of spirituality.

5. "Nonviolence."

6. Kelly Bulkeley, *Transforming Dreams: Learning Spiritual Lessons from the Dreams You Never Forget* (New York: John Wiley & Sons, 2000), 58.

7. *Tractatus* informs us of what can be said and what can only be shown (since it is outside the limit of language, it belongs to the realm of transcendence). The conflict between logic and our everyday existence as seen in the questions raised by traditional epistemologists emerges as a result of a misuse of language. In *Tractatus*, Wittgenstein mainly argues that there has to be a limit to thought.

8. Ludwig Wittgenstein, *Letters to Russell, Keynes, and Moore*, ed. G. H. von Wright (Ithaca, NY: Cornell University Press, 1974), 82. It was observed that, in order for him to redirect his thoughts from obsession, he would sit in the very first row of a theater. Russell Nieili, *Wittgenstein: From Mysticism to Ordinary Language* (New York: State University of New York Press, 1987), 166.

9. Bulkeley, *Transforming Dreams*, 62–63. It is interesting that according to Bulkeley, people who adjust well psychologically after experiencing trauma remember fewer dreams than those who do not adjust well. Further, dreams of well-adjusted people tend to be shorter, less complex, and less emotional.

10. Patricia O'Connell Killen and John de Beer, *The Art of Theological Reflection* (New York: Crossroad, 1994), x.

11. Rumi, *The Love Poems of Rumi*, ed. Deepak Chopra (New York: Harmony Books, 1998), 62.

12. In their study of the place of spirituality within the psychosocial adaptation of cancer patients, Andre Samson and Barbara Zerter affirm the centrality of the quest for meaning among these patients. Andre Samson and Barbara Zerter, "The Experience of Spirituality in the Psycho-Social Adaptation of Cancer Survivors," *The Journal of Pastoral Care & Counseling*, 57, no. 3 (2003): 339.

13. Blaise Pascal. *Pascal's Pensées* (New York: E. P. Dutton), 1958.

14. S. Radhakrishnan, *Indian Philosophy*, vol. 1 (Bombay: Blackie & Son, 1940), 589.

15. B. Bosanquet, *Contemporary Philosophy* (London: MacMillan, 1921), 57.

16. Cited by J. Wach, "Universals in Religion," in J. E. Smith, ed., *Philosophy of Religion* (New York: Macmillan, 1965), 85.

17. E. H. Cousin, "Models and the Future of Theology," in R. E. Whitson, *The Coming Convergence of World Religions* (New York: Newman, 1992), 188–200.

18. William James, *The Varieties of Religious Experience* (New York: Macmillan, 1961), 73.

19. R. Panikkar, *The Silence of God: The Answer of the Buddha*, trans. Robert Barr (New York: Orbis, 1989), 84.

20. R. Panikkar, *Myth, Faith, and Hermeneutics: Cross-Cultural Studies* (New York: Paulist Press, 1979), 4.

21. Ibid., 4. Panikkar's concept of myth as "collective consciousness" (*Myth, Faith, and Hermeneutics,* 52) is also reflected in the writing of Carl Jung. Describing Jung's collective consciousness, Sanford writes: "The collective unconscious is the sum total of the archetypes. It is the basic substratum of our psychic life." J. A. Sanford, *Dreams and Healing: A Succinct and Lively Interpretation of Dreams* (New York: Paulist Press, 1978), 17.

22. Panikkar, *Myth, Faith, and Hermeneutics,* 39.

23. In discussing the intuitive nature of understanding, Panikkar cites an Upanishadic saying: "Truth is understood with the heart; because, certainly, truth makes its home in the heart." Further along, he also quotes a Chinese teaching: "Just as big as the universal space is the space in the heart. In the heart lie heaven and earth, fire and wind, sun and moon, lightning and stars, what is and what is not; everything is contained in it." R. Panikkar, *A Dwelling Place for Wisdom* (Louisville, Kentucky: Westminster/John Knox, 1993), 17.

24. Panikkar, *Myth, Faith, and Hermeneutics*, 20.

25. See also Panikkar's description of "wisdom" as an integrative process in *A Dwelling Place for Wisdom,* 9.

26. Ibid., 92–93.

27. In referring to ontology, Tillich believes that, at the epistemological level, there is presupposed a subject-object interrelation between the subject (human beings) and the object (the world). This relationship makes the connection between the self and the world possible between the knowing subject and the known objects. Further, this subject-object relation manifests itself a priori. There is something in the structure of being, a priori, that speaks to the soul of human beings. Paul Tillich, *Systematic Theology*, vol. 1 (Chicago: University of Chicago Press, 1956) 163–171.

28. John P. Dourley, *The Psyche as Sacrament: A Comparative Study of C. G. Jung and Paul Tillich* (Toronto: Inner City Books, 1981), 19.

29. Tillich, *Systematic Theology*, vol. 1, 65.

30. F. J. Sheed, trans., *The Confessions of St. Augustine* (New York: Sheed & Ward, 1942), 3.

31. William James, *Varieties of Religious Experience* (New Hyde Park: University Books, 1963), 496.

32. Andrew Newberg, Eugene d'Aquili, and Vince Rause, *Why God Won't Go Away: Brain Science and the Biology of Belief* (New York: Ballantine, 2001), 7. See also A. Newberg, M. Pourdehnad, A. Alavis, E. d'Aquili, "Cerebral Blood Flow During Meditation: Preliminary Findings and Methodological Issues," *Perceptual Motor Skills* 97 (2003), 625–30.

Chapter Two

1. Brian P. Katz, *Myths of the World: Deities and Demons of the Far East* (New York: Metrobooks, 1995), 85–86.

2. Paul Tillich, *Theology of Culture* (New York: Oxford University Press, 1959), 47–51.

3. Katz, *Myths of the World*, 58. According to the myth, the goddess Amaterasu hid herself in the cave to avoid the foolish behaviors and practical jokes of her brother Susanowo, the storm god. Then the world grew dim and the evil spirits roamed around the earth. The other deities, recognizing the situation, got together to try to coax the sun goddess to come out. They danced and sang, and out of curiosity, Amaterasu peeked out of her cave and asked Uzume what was happening. Uzume told her that there was a more supreme god than her Augustness. When Amaterasu asked who, Uzume presented a mirror. While trying to find out what was happening, the other deities blocked the entrance to the cave.

4. Ibid., 93.

5. Both were incarnations of Lord Vishnu.

6. Anthony Christie, *Chinese Mythology* (Italy: Hymlyn Publishing, 1968), 55–56.

7. Ibid., 92.

8. Leslie Marmon Silko, *Ceremony* (New York: Penguin, 1986), 2.

9. Andrew Newberg, Eugene d'Aquili, and Vince Rause, *Why God Won't Go Away: Brain Science and the Biology of Belief* (New York: Ballantine, 2001), 67–72.

10. Ann and Barry Ulanov recognize the role religion plays in providing containment for individuals. In her words, true containment "gives primordial experience a place and a state of being in which it finds itself at ease with us and we find ourselves at ease with it." *Religion and the Unconscious* (Philadelphia: Westminster Press, 1975), 25. In a similar fashion, myth offers a safe space for our primordial experiences and thus enables the soul to find a resting place.

11. Newberg, d'Aquili, and Rause, *Why God Won't Go Away*, 69.

12. Niels Mulder, *Everyday Life in Thailand: An Interpretation* (Bangkok: Duang Kamol, 1979), 27.

13. *Saksit* may be translated "sacred."

14. Mulder, *Everyday Life in Thailand*, 28.

15. Ibid., 33.

16. Teik Beng Tan, *Beliefs and Practices Among Malaysian Chinese Buddhists* (Kuala Lumpur: Buddhist Missionary Society, 1988), 66–68.

17. Roger Schmidt et al., "Tribal Religions in Historical Times," in *Patterns of Religion* (Belmont, CA: Wadsworth, 1999), 134.

18. Newberg, d'Aquili, and Rause, *Why God Won't Go Away*, 85.

19. Tillich, *Theology of Culture*, 54.

20. John Shelby Spong, *A New Christianity for a New World: Why Traditional Faith Is Dying and How a New Faith Is Being Born* (San Francisco: HarperSanFrancisco, 2001), 11.

21. Ibid., 3–4.

Chapter Three

1. Roger Schmidt et al., "Tribal Religions in Historical Times," in *Patterns of Religion* (Belmont, CA: Wadsworth, 1999), 9.

2. Sheldon Cashdan, *Object Relations Therapy: Using the Relationship* (New York: W. W. Norton, 1988), 33.

3. It is translated as "desire" or "want."

4. Pamela Lee Cranton, "Kaddish Poem," *The Journal of Pastoral Care & Counseling* 57, no. 1 (2003): 98.

5. Siroj Sorajjakool and Bryn Seyle, "Theological Strategies, Constructed Meaning, and Coping with Breast Cancer: A Qualitative Study," *Pastoral Psychology* 54, no.2 (2005): 173–86.

6. Patricia Fryack and Bonita Reinert, "Spirituality and People with Potentially Fatal Diagnoses," *Nursing Forum* 34, no. 1 (1999): 20.

7. Genesis 32:24–28, New International Version.

Chapter Four

1. Rabindranath Tagore, *Gitanjali: A Collection of Prose Translations Made by the Author from the Original Bengali* (New York: Scribner Poetry, 1941), 102.

2. Patricia O'Connell Killen and John de Beer, *The Art of Theological Reflection* (New York: Crossroad, 1994), x.

3. Judith Lewis Herman, *Trauma and Recovery: The Aftermath of Violence from Domestic Abuse and Political Terror* (New York: Basic Books, 1992), 41.

4. Rachel Naomi Remen, *My Grandfather's Blessings: Stories of Strength, Refuge, and Belonging* (New York: Riverhead Books, 2000), 28–29.

5. Antti Oksanen, *Religious Conversion: A Meta-Analysis Study* (Sweden: Lund University Press, 1994), 84.

6. C. Ullman, "Cognitive and Emotional Antecedents of Religious Conversion," *Journal of Personality and Social Psychology* 43, no. 1 (1982): 183–92.

7. S. Syrjanen, "In Search of Meaning and Identity: Conversion to Christianity in Pakistani Muslim Culture," *Annals of the Finnish Society of Missiology and Ecumenics* 45 (1984): 90. According to this study, nine lost one or both of their parents when they were young, ten had problems with their parents, six experienced guilt and restlessness, eight had economic difficulties, three experienced alienation, and three had other problems. For more in-depth studies on conversion, see Antti Oksanen, *Religious Conversion: A Meta-Analysis*.

8. Andre Samson and Barbara Zerter, "The Experience of Spirituality in the Psycho-Social Adaptation of Cancer Survivors," *The Journal of Pastoral Care & Counseling* 57, no. 3 (2003): 334.

9. Ibid., 339.

10. Elizabeth Johnston Taylor, "Spiritual Needs of Patients with Cancer and Family Caregivers," *Cancer Nursing* 26, no. 4 (2003): 265.

11. Kristen Leslie, *When Violence Is No Stranger: Pastoral Counseling with Survivors of Acquaintance Rape* (Minneapolis: Augsburg Fortress, 2003), 100.

12. Elizabeth Kubler-Ross, *On Death and Dying: What the Dying Have to Teach Doctors, Nurses, Clergy, and Their Own Families* (New York: Collier, 1969).

13. Henri Nouwen, *Lifesigns: Intimacy, Fecundity, and Ecstasy in Christian Perspective* (New York: Image Books, 1966), 99.

14. Marja Ohman, Siv Soderberg, and Berit Lundman, "Hovering Between Suffering and Enduring: The Meaning of Living with Serious Chronic Illness," *Qualitative Health Research* 13, no. 4 (April 2003): 540.

15. Siroj Sorajjakool, "Getting There Without Going Anywhere: Chuang Tzu's Nothingness and Spiritual Transformation" (2003), 53. Unpublished manuscript.

16. At the age of fourteen, his son died of progeria, a rare disease that speeds up the victim's aging. Kristin E. Holmes, "23rd Psalm Holds Answers to Many of Life's Questions," *The Riverside Press-Enterprise*, October 25, 2005, B12.

17. Ibid.

18. Ibid.

19. David Karp, *Speaking of Sadness: Depression, Disconnection, and the Meanings of Illness* (Oxford: Oxford University Press, 1996).

20. Johnny Ramirez-Johnson, Carlos Fayard, Carlos Garberoglio, and Clara M. Jorge Ramirez, "Is Faith an Emotion? Faith as a Meaning-Making Affective Process: An Example from Breast Cancer Patients," *American Behavioral Scientist* 45, no. 12 (August 2002): 1839–53.

21. Jenenne Nelson, "Struggling to Gain Meaning: Living with the Uncertainty of Breast Cancer," *Advances in Nursing Science* 18, no. 3 (March 1996): 59–76.

22. Siroj Sorajjakool and Bryn Seyle, "Theological Strategies, Constructed Meaning, and Coping with Breast Cancer: A Qualitative Study" *Pastoral Psychology* 54, no.2, (2005): 173–86.

23. Ibid.

24. Siroj Sorajjakool, Kelvin Thompson, Leigh Aveling, and Art Earll, "Chronic Pain, Meaning, and Spirituality: A Qualitative Study of the Healing Process in Relation to the Role of Meaning Among Individuals with Chronic Pain" (accepted for publication by *The Journal of Pastoral Care & Counseling*, February 2005). The concept of reformulation of the self in a healing process is also expressed by J. Morse and B. Carter, "The Essence of Enduring and Expressions of Suffering: The Reformulation of Self," *Scholarly Inquiry for Nursing Practice* 10 (1996): 43–60. According to Andre Samson and Barbara Zerter, healing takes place through a broader understanding of themselves, others, and the world. Samson and Zerter, "The Experience of Spirituality in the Psycho-Social Adaptation of Cancer Survivors," 341.

25. Siroj Sorajjakool, "Thai Women's Experiences with AIDS: Perspectives on Religion and Coping" (accepted for publication by *Journal of HIV/AIDS and Social Services*, forthcoming, 2006).

26. Albert Y. Hsu, *Grieving a Suicide: A Loved One's Search for Comfort, Answers and Hope* (Urbana, IL: InterVarsity Press, 2002), 89.

27. Jory Graham, *In the Company of Others: Understanding the Human Needs of Cancer Patients* (New York: Harcourt Brace Jovanovich, 1982), 21–22.

Chapter Five

1. Paul Tillich, *Systematic Theology*, vol. 2 (London: SCM, 1957), 125–35.

2. Ibid., 126.

3. Paul Tillich, *The Courage to Be* (London: Fount Paperbacks, 1952), 152.

4. John Macquarrie, *Principles of Christian Theology* (New York: Charles Scribner's Sons, 1966), 236.

5. Ibid., 447.

6. Ibid., 452.

7. Dietrich Bonhoeffer, *Letters and Papers from Prison* (New York: McMillan, 1971), 360.

8. R. Panikkar, *Myth, Faith, and Hermeneutics: Cross-Cultural Studies* (New York: Paulist Press, 1979), 262.

9. Ibid., 264.

10. Ibid., 265.

11. Ibid., 273.

12. Ibid., 390.

13. Ibid., 39.

14. Raimundo Panikkar, *The Silence of God: The Answer of the Buddha* (New York: Orbis, 1989), 84.

15. Panikkar, *Myth, Faith, and Hermeneutics*, 403.

16. Ibid., 406.

17. Ibid., 413.

18. Ibid., 434.

19. Ibid., 454.

20. Ibid., 437.

21. Yu-lan Feng, *A Short History of Chinese Philosophy: A Systematic Account of Chinese Thought from Its Origin to the Present Day* (New York: Free Press, 1948), 221.

22. Ibid. 221.

23. Ann Ulanov, "Chaos, Consciousness, and Plenum," *Journal of Religion and Health* 39, no. 3 (2000): 208.

24. Cited by Fritjof Capra, *The Tao of Physics* (New York: Bantam Books, 1983), 131.

25. Ibid., 131.

26. Cited by Wing-Tsit Chan, *The Source Book in Chinese Philosophy* (Princeton, NJ: Princeton University Press, 1963), 140.

27. Ibid., 136.

28. Siroj Sorajjakool, *Wu Wei, Negativity, and Depression: The Principle of Non-Trying in the Practice of Pastoral Care* (New York: Haworth Pastoral Press, 2001), 81–86.

29. Friedrich Nietzsche, *Thus Spoke Zarathustra*, trans. Walter Kaufmann, in *The Portable Nietzsche* (New York: Penguin Books, 1954), 157.

30. "Mother Goddess as Kali–The Feminine Force in Indian Art" (August 2000): 7, http://www.exoticindiaart.com/kali.htm.

31. Carl Jung, *Psychology and Alchemy*, trans. R. F. C Hull (London: Routledge & Kegan Paul, 1953), 217–21.

32. There are three stages, according to Jung, in the alchemical process individuals need to go through. *Nigredo* (darkness or blackening) is the first stage of individuation. It is the recognition and integration of our shadow aspects that have been repressed out of consciousness into the personal unconscious from where they reappear via dreams or projections onto others. The work of alchemy begins with mass *confusa* or *prima materia*, composed of four common base metals: lead, tin, copper, and iron. In psychological terms, it refers to opposite elements within a person's unconscious mind. These opposite qualities are often undifferentiated and disintegrated. In this process, the alchemist heats the material in order to reduce it to a state of fine powder. When it is putrefied, it begins to separate. The final state of *negredo* is the distillation process—the boiling of the liquid and reconverting the vapor into a liquid again by cooling it. Jung, *Psychology of Alchemy*, 261–62. See also Thom F. Cavalli, *Alchemical Psychology: Old Recipes for Living in a New World* (New York: Putnam, 2002), 180–81. This entire process represents the process of individuation. It represents the (a) integration of the shadow and recognition of the opposites within us; (b)

heating refers to the emotional outburst that causes us to reflect on ourselves, what it is within us that drives us to such behavior; (c) putrefaction, the separation of the shadow aspects from each other, the beginning of recognition; and (d) the solution refers to refinements of the shadow—cleansing via the process of bringing the shadow into consciousness. *Albedo* (the whitening phase) is the stage when the alchemist seeks to keep an even and regular temperature in order to make certain the mixture doesn't overheat. This helps dry the ingredients and allows them to cool down and return to the basic black mass. In psychological terms, it represents the first transmutation and integration of the inner contra-sexual components, the anima in the man and the animus in the woman. (See Cavalli, *Alchemical Psychology*, 181–83.) *Rubedo* (red) is the last procedure in the work of alchemy. According to Aristotle, "the philosopher's stone (red) is the grand finale of the system—the final cause that can reproduce itself." At this stage a reconciliation of the opposites occurs and in so doing, the self (and all elements that used to reside in the unconscious) is brought into being or consciousness (see Cavalli, *Alchemical Psychology*, 183–85.)

Chapter Six

1. Anton T. Boisen, *Out of the Depths: An Autobiographical Study of Mental Disorder and Religious Experience* (New York: Harper & Bros., 1960), 95.

2. Ibid., 204–5.

3. Arthur Osborne, *Ramana Maharishi and the Path of Self-Knowledge* (New York: Samuel Weiser, 1954), 35–36.

4. Raymond H. Prince, "Religious Experience and Psychopathology: Cross-Cultural Perspectives," in *Religion and Mental Health*, ed. John F. Schumaker (New York: Oxford, 1992), 281–90.

5. Henry James Sr., *Substance and Shadow* (Boston: Ticknor & Fields, 1863), 75, cited in Kay R. Jamison, *Touched with Fire: Manic-Depressive Illness and the Artistic Temperament* (New York: Free Press, 1996), 207.

6. Martha Manning, *Undercurrents: A Life Beneath the Surface* (San Francisco: HarperSanFrancisco, 1994), 101.

7. Gerald May, *Simply Sane: The Spirituality of Mental Health* (New York: Crossroad, 1977), 45.

8. Arthur Kleinman, "How Is Culture Important for DSM-IV?" in *Culture and Psychiatric Diagnosis: A DSM-IV Perspective*, ed. Juan E. Mezzich, Arthur Kleinman, Horacio Fabrega Jr., and Delores L. Parron (Washington, D.C.: American Psychiatric Press, 1996), 17.

9. Ibid., 18.

10. Ibid., 19.

11. Michel Foucault, *Mental Illness and Psychology* (Berkeley: University of California Press, 1962), 63.

12. Anthony J. Marsella, Norman Sartorius, Assen Jablensky, and Fred R. Fenton, "Cross-Cultural Studies of Depressive Disorders: An Overview," in *Culture and Depression: Studies in the Anthropology and Cross-Cultural Psychiatry of Affect and Disorder*, ed. Arthur Kleinman and Byron Good (Berkeley: University of California Press, 1985), 305.

13. Ibid., 306.

14. Kleinman, "How is Culture Important for DSM-IV?" 17–18.

15. Rachel T. Harre-Mustin and Jeanne Marecek, "Abnormal and Clinical Psychology: The Politics of Madness," in *Critical Psychology: An Introduction*, ed. Dennis Fox and Isaac Prilleltensky (Longon: Sage, 1997), 108. Another interesting example of the politics of psychology is the IQ test. Researchers such as Leon Kamin and Stephen Gould believe that the pioneers of intelligence testing were motivated by social agendas as well as by scientific endeavors, that they believed in the "genetic inferiority of immigrants, Blacks, Native Americans, Jews, and women." This prejudicial perspective extended into the realm of social policies as well, affecting the immigration laws of the 1920s, thus prohibiting Eastern European Jews to enter the United States in the 1930s. It also led to the involuntary sterilization laws passed by many states to stop the spread of feeble-mindedness. Benjamin Harris, "Repoliticizing the History of Psychology," in *Critical Psychology*, 25–28.

16. Foucault, *Mental Illness and Psychology*, 62.

17. Hubert Dreyfus, "Foreword," *Mental Illness and Psychology*, xxvi.

18. Cited by Dreyfus, ibid.

19. Robert Hedaya, *Understanding Biological Psychiatry* (New York: W. W. Norton, 1996), 67.

20. Neuromodulation refers to the process that causes changes in the structure and function of the nerve cell and the growth of new connections between nerve cells. It is responsible for changes in short-term and long-term learning, memory, and change. Ibid., 33–34.

21. Ibid., 69. Areas most often affected by sensitization and kindling are the hippocampus and the limbic system.

22. Carl Jung, *Psychology and Western Religion*, trans. R. F. C. Hull (Princeton: Princeton University Press, 1984), 202.

23. Thomas Moore, *Care of the Soul: A Guide for Cultivating Depth and Sacredness in Everyday Life* (New York: HarperPerennial, 1992), 137–38.

24. Ibid., 21.

25. What we often do not recognize about our shadow, according to Jung, is that it also contains idealized traits that have been repressed, and we can describe these positive traits as heroic, visionary, spiritual, vital, noble, and refined. It contains the positive instinctive qualities that we have been repressing for one reason or another. For example, if a person wants to make his or her mark in this modern world, he or she has to go all out. In order to do this, he or she may neglect certain values in his or her life. An artistic person may neglect and repress his or her artistic instinct since it does not seem to help he or she achieve his or her goals in the business world. But the gift of art is placed there by God, and God will continually remind us about it. Either the artist will come back and pick up this aspect of their nature or they will stagnate spiritually and emotionally.

26. Gerald May, *Simply Sane: The Spirituality of Mental Health* (New York: Crossroad, 1977), 130.

Chapter Seven

1. Søren Kierkegaard, *Parables of Kierkegaard*, ed. Thomas C. Oden (Princeton, NJ: Princeton University Press, 1978), 87.

2. Although he was buried in the family plot, because of the jealousy of his

brother, the bishop of Aalborg, there is no sign to indicate where his body lies.

3. Walter Lowrie, *A Short Life of Kierkegaard* (Princeton, NJ: Princeton University Press, 1942), 18.

4. On December 4, 1780, when he was twenty-four, he obtained a license to deal with foodstuffs. On September 19, 1788, he was licensed to deal in Chinese and East India wares as well as with merchandise from the Danish West Indies (sugar, syrup, and coffee beans). In his early thirties he became a wholesale grocer on a big scale. Ibid., 21.

5. His early retirement was caused, most probably, by the sudden death of his first wife.

6. In *Point of View*, Kierkegaard writes: "As a child I was strictly and austerely brought up in Christianity; humanly speaking, crazily brought up. A child crazily travestied as a melancholy old man. Terrible!" (Søren Kierkegaard, *Point of View* [Princeton, NJ: Princeton University Press, 1998]).

7. Lowrie, *Short Life of Kierkegaard*, 24. Søren Kierkegaard describes his father as "the most melancholy man I have ever known."

8. His father may have chosen the time when Søren was twenty-five years old, when according to Danish law he came of age, to confess his sin to his son.

9. Some sort of paralysis was believed to be the result. During one of the social gatherings, he fell and lay helpless on the floor. He asked his friends not to pick "it" up but to "leave it" there till the maid comes in the morning to sweep. Lowrie, *Short Life of Kierkegaard*, 41.

10. Ibid., 42.

11. The reason for his starting a journal is explained when he writes: "The apparent wealth of thoughts and ideas one is sensible of in the abstract possibility must be just as uncomfortable and evoke the same sort of unrest as the cows suffer from when they are not milked at the proper time." Ibid., 61.

12. This secret of his father was retold in the story of Antigone (a female character); see Søren Kierkegaard, *Either/Or: A Fragment of Life* (New York: Penguin Classics, 1992).

13. Cited by Walter Lowrie, *Short Life of Kierkegaard*, 80.

14. Ibid., 82.

15. His journal reveals that he was very attracted to this principle.

16. Lowrie, *Short Life of Kierkegaard*, 97.

17. Kierkegaard writes: "One blows one's brains out, bing, bang, bover, then the story is over; and snip, snap, snother, now can begin another." "One who went out and thought of committing suicide—at the same instant a stone fell down and killed him, and he ended with the words, 'God be praised.'" Ibid., 99.

18. According to P. A. Heilberg's construction, Kierkegaard was led by a group of boon companions to "one of those places where, strangely enough, one gives money for a woman's despicableness." This statement is recorded in a story called "A Possibility." Ibid., 100.

19. This "reformation" went very slowly. Kierkegaard repeated this very same statement about a year later. Ibid., 105.

20. Ibid., 114. According to Lowrie, Kierkegaard was several times "on the verge" of insanity and often meditated suicide during his revolt and defiance against his father and God. Ibid., 27.

21. Ibid., 107.

22. Ibid., 108.

23. Ibid., 121.

24. "I am a penitent" was Kierkegaard's frequent remark to his acquaintances.

25. Lowrie, *Short Life of Kierkegaard*, 124.

26. In describing himself in relation to the breaking of his engagement, Kierkegaard writes: "About me there is something rather ghostly, which accounts for the fact that no one can put up with me who has to see me in everyday intercourse and so comes into real relationship." Ibid., 140.

27. He believed that marriage called for total honesty but he could not see himself being able to open himself up totally regarding his father's curse and sensuality. This struggle is recorded in *Either/Or*, where Antigone could not reveal the secret that would bring disgrace to her father.

28. Josiah Thompson, *Kierkegaard* (New York: Alfred A. Knopf, 1973), 116.

29. Ibid., 128.

30. The *Corsair* was a comic paper founded by Aaron Goldschmidt. It was cleverly managed and had attained the biggest circulation in Denmark because of its unremitting ridicule directed at Copenhagen's nobles.

31. Thompson, *Kierkegaard*, 190. Even after the *Corsair* ceased to exist, the name Søren had become comic through the whole of Scandinavia. No parents would name their children Søren (Lowrie, *Short Life of Kierkegaard*, 180).

32. Søren Kierkegaard, *Journals of Kierkegaard*, ed. Alexander Dru (New York: Harper, 1958), 127–28.

33. Lowrie, *Short Life of Kierkegaard*, 201.

34. Kierkegaard, *Journals of Kierkegaard*, 137–38.

35. Ibid., 142.

36. In describing this experience, Kierkegaard recorded in his journal in 1852: "Then came 1848. I was lifted up to a height which I had never before known, and perfectly understood myself in what had gone before, and the past." Ibid., 215. This event was described by Lowrie as a "radical cure," in that after this incident, Kierkegaard never again resorted to the use of pseudonyms. Lowrie, *Short Life of Kierkegaard*, 208.

37. Lowrie, *Short Life of Kierkegaard*, 208.

38. Kierkegaard, *Journals of Kierkegaard*, 217.

39. In describing himself as a little pinch of spice, he writes: "A little pinch of spice! Humanly speaking, what a painful thing to be thus sacrificed, to be the little pinch of spice! But on the other hand God knows well the man whom He elects to employ in this way, and so He also knows how, in the inward understanding of it, to make it so blessed a thing for him to be sacrificed, that among the thousands of divers voices which express, each in its own way, the same thing, his also will be heard, and perhaps especially his, which is truly de profundis, proclaiming: God is love . . . But underneath all these sopranos, supporting them as it were, as the bass part does, is audible the de profundis which issues from the sacrificed one: God is love." Lowrie, *Short Life of Kierkegaard*, 260.

40. In modern time the illness kills 14 percent of its victims. When the lung membrane is attacked by this infection, the germs remain in constant movement as the patient breathes, so that even if the infection subsides, it never gets a chance to heal. The patient coughs unremittingly and finally dies of infection and exhaustion. Thompson, *Kierkegaard*, 231. According to the hospital record, he continued to cough and "The expectorate consists of purulent clots,

a few of which are closely mixed with light red blood." His heart rate averaged at 100–130 per minute and his strength decreased visibly. *Kierkegaard: Letters and Documents* (Princeton, NJ: Princeton University Press, 1978), 28–33. See also Henning Fenger, *Kierkegaard, the Myths and Their Origins: Studies in the Kierkegaardian Papers and Letters*, trans. George C. Schoolfield (New Haven: Yale University Press, 1980), 66.

41. Kierkegaard sees the ethical realm as an arena for one to achieve actuality. This concept is closely related to Fitche's Ego, empirical ego (man) and non-empirical ego (external world), where the non-empirical ego is the arena for empirical ego to perform moral duty. W. K. Wright, *A History of Modern Philosophy* (New York: Macmillan, 1941), 298–305.

42. Søren Kierkegaard, *Fear and Trembling* and *Sickness Unto Death* (Princeton, NJ: Princeton University Press, 1954), 150–51.

43. Kierkegaard, *Journals of Kierkegaard*, 190.

44. Lowrie, *Short Life of Kierkegaard*, 76.

45. Kierkegaard, *Journals of Kierkegaard*, 139–40.

46. Ibid., 215.

47. Ibid., 217.

Chapter Eight

1. Cited in Kosuke Koyama, *Waterbuffalo Theology* (New York: Orbis, 1974), 205.

2. Richards and Bergin offer five reasons why spiritual assessment is essential, particularly in a therapeutic relationship. First, understanding clients' worldviews can help one become more empathetic and sensitive. Second, it can increase an understanding of how healthy or unhealthy a client's spiritual orientation is and to what extent it affects the presenting problem. Third, to see if the beliefs and the community can be used as resources for clients' coping methods and growth. Fourth, to find out which spiritual interventions are beneficial for the client. And lastly, to determine if there are unresolved spiritual issues. Based on these reasons, they propose nine dimensions that should be included in the process of assessment: metaphysical worldview, religious affiliation, religious orthodoxy (the extent to which one adheres to one's doctrinal beliefs), religious problem-solving style (three coping styles are: self-directing: a person resolves his or her own problems; deferring: a person defers his or her problems to God; and collaborative: the responsibility is held jointly between a person and his or her God), spiritual identity, God image, value-lifestyle congruence, doctrinal knowledge, and religious and spiritual health and maturity. P. Scott Richards and Allen E. Bergin, *A Spiritual Strategy for Counseling and Psychotherapy* (Washington, D.C.: American Psychological Association, 1997), 172–87.

3. Dietrich Bonhoeffer, *Letters and Papers from Prison* (New York: McMillan, 1971), 361.

4. Ibid., 369–70.

5. James W. Fowler, *Stages of Faith: The Psychology of Human Development and the Quest for Meaning* (San Francisco: Harper & Row, 1981), 198. Fowler proposes six stages in faith development: (1) intuitive-projective faith: faith dominated by ego-centricism. An individual assumes that everyone should understand God the same way; (2) mythic-literal faith: a stage of literal interpretation

of stories. An individual often believes that God wants what that individual wants; (3) synthetic-conventional faith: a strong need for group approval and approval from significant others. An individual tends to seek compliance with social and religious norms; (4) individuative-reflective faith: an individual search for truth that moves beyond convention. An individual finds that what was taught does not make sense and has to make an individual search to make sense of things for him- or herself; (5) conjunctive faith (as stated in the chapter); and (6) universalizing faith: a rare stage of sainthood. They live in this world and yet are unaffected by the world. They often may not be appreciated by the world of their time because their beliefs and ideas transcend the ordinary.

6. Lao Tzu, *Tao Te Ching*, trans. Stephen Mitchell (New York: HarperPerennial, 1988), 1.

7. Chuang Tzu, *Chuang Tzu: Basic Writings*, trans. Burton Watson (New York: Columbia University Press, 1996), 40.

8. R. Panikkar, *The Silence of God: The Answer of the Buddha;* trans. Robert Barr (New York: Orbis, 1989). See also Panikkar's *Myth, Faith, and Hermeneutics: Cross-Cultural Studies* (New York: Paulist Press, 1979), 4.

9. J. Krishnamurti, *In the Light of Silence All Problems Are Dissolved* (Chennai: Krishnamurti Foundation India, 1992), 54.

10. Hinduism proposes four stages of development. For students, the aim is to acquire information and cultivate habits for the formation of good character. The marriage stage is when one starts a family, plans for the future, becomes responsible, strives for success, and participates in the life of the community. The retirement stage is when one needs to work out one's own personal philosophy and strive to understand the meaning of life that transcends material possessions or the external world. The final stage, *sanyasin*, is one who neither hates nor loves anything. He is unaffected by external forces.

11. This is a part of a song written by Swami Vevekananda called "Song of *Sannyasin*," quoted from http://kaustubh88.tripod.com/sos.html.

12. Koenig, *Spirituality in Patient Care* (Philadelphia: Templeton Foundation Press, 2001), 22. Other useful modalities include: Kuhn's Spiritual Inventory developed by Clifford Kuhn of the University of Louisville's psychiatry department. This model looks at seven areas (meaning, belief, love, forgiveness, prayer, meditation, and worship); Matthews' Spiritual History developed by Dale Matthews of Georgetown University. This tool asks three basic questions addressing the importance of religion, the possible influence of beliefs on medical care, and patients' openness to explore spirituality; the FICA Spiritual Assessment Tool was developed by Christina Puchalski at George Washington University. "F" stands for faith, "I" for important, "C" for church, "A" for apply and address (as in addressing spiritual needs); Maugans' SPIRITual History was developed by Todd Maugans of the family medicine department at the University of Virginia. "S" stands for spiritual beliefs, "P" for personal spirituality, "I" for integration within the community, "R" for rituals, "I" for implications for medical care, and "T" for terminal events planning; The HOPE Questionnaire was developed by Gowri Anandarajah and Ellen Hight of the family medicine department at Brown University. It looks at the source of hope and meaning, the place of organized religion, personal spirituality and how it is being practiced, and effects on medical care and end-of-life issues. See Koenig, *Spirituality in Patient Care*, 88–94.

13. Richard L. Gorsuch and William Miller, "Assessing Spirituality," in *Inte-*

grating Spirituality into Treatment: Resources for Practitioners, ed. William Miller (Washington, D.C.: American Psychological Association, 1999), 52–53.

14. In her qualitative study of spiritual needs of patients with cancer, Elizabeth Johnston Taylor, associate professor of nursing at Loma Linda University, finds that one of the questions emerging from spirituality issues among cancer patients is the "Why" question: "Why me/us? Or why not me? Or what did I/we do to deserve this?" Elizabeth Johnston Taylor, "Spiritual Needs of Patients with Cancer and Family Caregivers," *Cancer Nursing* 26, no. 4 (2003): 265. Fintel and McDermott, in *Dear God, It's Cancer*, suggest that there are three answers to the why question that seem to bring peace and meaning to patients. These are: cancer is a test from God, cancer is God's way of turning us to him, and cancer is God's way of making us better people. William A. Fintel and Gerald R. McDermott, *Dear God, It's Cancer: A Medical and Spiritual Guide for Patients and Their Families* (Dallas: Word Publishing, 1997), 181–98.

15. Fintel and McDermott, *Dear God, It's Cancer*, 181.

16. Ethel S. Person, *By Force of Fantasy: How We Make Our Lives* (New York: Basic Books, 1995), 37.

17. Koyama, *Waterbuffalo Theology*, 206.

18. Ibid., 208.

Chapter Nine

1. Rachel Naomi Remen, *My Grandfather's Blessings: Stories of Strength, Refuge, and Belonging* (New York: Riverhead Books, 2000), 199.

2. Friedrich Nietzsche, "Schopenhauer as Educator," in *Unmodern Observations*, ed. William Arrowsmith (New Haven: Yale University Press, 1990), 165.

3. James E. Dittes, *Pastoral Counseling: The Basics* (Louisville: Westminster John Knox, 1999), 57.

4. Stephen Muse, "The Meaning of Psychotherapy," *Journal of Pastoral Care* 52, no. 2 (1998): 186.

5. Thomas Moore, *Care of the Soul: A Guide for Cultivating Depth and Sacredness in Everyday Life* (New York: HarperPerennial, 1992), xv.

6. Henry Nouwen, *Lifesigns: Intimacy, Fecundity, and Ecstasy in Christian Perspective* (New York: Doubleday, 1989), 27. Erik Erikson calls this place the "in-between state" that offers synthetic function of the ego, thus enhancing the state of health and wholeness. *Identity and the Life Cycle* (New York: W. W. Norton, 1980), 23–25.

7. Nouwen, *Lifesigns*, 38–39.

8. Ibid., 71.

9. Ibid.

10. Ann Belford Ulanov, *Finding Space: Winnicott, God, and Psychic Reality* (Louisville, KY: Westminster John Knox, 2001), 33–34.

11. Ibid., 37. Ulanov's subjective-object God-images refer to the subjective understanding of God through our imagination. The objective-object God is the God who stands in the tradition of our faith outside of our subjective feelings. The objective-subject refers to the God out there (objectively real) who is in touch with our subjective experiences.

12. D. W. Winnicott, *Playing and Reality* (London: Routledge, 1971), 41.

13. Dittes, *Pastoral Counseling*, 61.

14. Elisabeth Kubler-Ross, *On Death and Dying: What the Dying Have to*

Teach Doctors, Nurses, Clergy, and Their Own Families (New York: Collier, 1969), 35.

15. Ibid., 36.

16. Ibid., 41.

17. Allison Nichols, "A Little More About Prayer," *Journal of Pastoral Care* 54, no. 4 (2000): 469–70.

18. Ibid., 70.

19. Jewel Kilcher, *A Night Without Armor* (New York: HarperCollins, 1999), 135.

Appendix 2

1. *Prajapati* literally refers to the Lord of the creatures. The concept of *Prajapati* signifies an important shift from henotheism to monotheism in the development of Hindu religious thinking. S. Radhakrishnan, *Indian Philosophy,* vol. 1 (Bombay: Blackie & Son, 1940), 90–92.

2. R. Panikkar, *Myth, Faith, and Hermeneutics: Cross-Cultural Studies* (New York: Paulist Press, 1979), 32.

3. Ibid., 45.

4. Panikkar is not against reason as much as he wants to keep reason in its proper place. In the realm of morality, reason cannot be the ground for our conduct. Reason is rather a tool. We often use reason to seek justification of the self. To seek this justification is to set oneself higher than God. It is to suggest that my reason (and even my reasoning about God) is the basis of my conduct. The creature's role is to obey. For this reason, the creature's function is not to find out whether what he or she does is good or bad but rather "to do" and to act out of obedience with reason as a tool. In discussing obedience, Panikkar states: "I obey not because I see the rationale of the commandment, . . . but because I see I must obey, (ibid., 55). For discussion of a similar concept, see Bonhoeffer's *Ethics*, where he proposes that the first task of Christian ethics is to overcome the knowledge of good and evil. Dietrich Bonhoeffer, *Ethics* (New York: Macmillan, 1965).

5. Panikkar, *Myth, Faith, and Hermeneutics*, 67.

6. Ibid., 83.

7. Panikkar, *A Dwelling Place for Wisdom* (Louisville, Kentucky: Westminster/John Knox, 1993), 14. The relation between myth and wisdom is reflected in his usage of the quotation by Heraclitus: "Only one thing is wise, to recognize the insight which directs everything through everything." Ibid., 9.

8. The three mythemes from the myth of *Sunahsepa* described by Panikkar are: (1) presence of death: life is a constant confrontation with death. Facing death is a part of human condition; (2) solidarity of life: life is not private property. It is something we share with the living. "We live only because we bear and express this supra-individual life." We are called to lead this spatio-temporal individual into the transcendental supra-individual life; and (3) transcendental desire: this desire reflects that deep within the core of our being resides a desire for true authenticity that goes beyond the bondage of the encapsulated self within the realm of materialism and social status. Or, in Jungian terms, it is the desire for full individuation (the fully differentiated self). *Myth, Faith, and Hermeneutics*, 155–62.

9. Ibid., 159.

10. Ibid.

11. Ibid.

12. Ibid., 160.

13. Paul Tillich, *The Courage to Be* (London: Collins, 1952), 48–49.

14. Panikkar. *Myth, Faith, and Hermeneutics*, 160.

15. Ibid., 160.

16. In this ancient myth recorded in the Rg Veda, Sunahsepa is being offered as a sacrifice by his own father Ajigarta, so that this sacrifice can spare the life of Rohita and his father, King Hariscandra. Panikkar. *Myth, Faith, and Hermeneutics,* 105–25

17. Panikkar, *Myth, Faith, and Hermeneutics*, 172.

18. This concept also finds expression in Tillich's understanding of the authentic self that takes place when the self is able to overcome the fear and anxiety of death and meaninglessness. This ability to overcome is phrased "the courage to be," which finds its fullest expression in Jesus Christ, who conquered death boldly. See *The Courage to Be*.

19. This is a turning away of human beings from God toward self. It is not a conscious turning away as much as it is an ontological state of being. When we ask for God, we have already been estranged from God. In the moral realm, the laws that we need suggest that we are not united with God in will and therefore need laws to govern us.

20. Hubris or self-elevation. This is when we make ourselves the center and not God. We make ourselves the center because of our awareness of infinity and our unwillingness to admit our finitude (metaphysically we want to claim absolute truth; in morality we want to identify with absolute goodness; in culture we identify our creations with divine creativity).

21. The striving for hunger, power, and sex leads to human estrangement. This does not end because human desire in the estranged state is insatiable. In an essential state, the desire is always a desire to be united with the object of one's love for its own sake. It becomes concupiscence when it seeks pleasure for itself.

22. Early in his career, Jung recognized the irreducible nature of the psyche's religious function. Through his clinical experience, Jung discovered materials that correspond to dogmas, creeds, and religious symbols. They may be classified in three categories: (1) An examination of neurosis. Jung observed that most illnesses, especially in patients over thirty-five, are the result of loss of religious meaning. Neurosis refers to the suffering of human beings who have not discovered the meaning of life; (2) The appearance of dream images. Jung discovers the appearance of dream images that arouse a sense of fear and awe in the dreamer and thus make the person feel in touch with transpersonal meaning. These dream images often correspond to aspects of religious creeds; (3) The process of individuation. This shows that a goal of wholeness is integral to the psyche. Inherent in the drive to wholeness is the production of symbols that fulfill and reconcile opposing polarities of the psyche. These symbols depict images of God.

23. Ann Ulanov and Barry Ulanov, *Religion and the Unconscious*, (Philadelphia: Westminster Press, 1975), 35.

24. Ibid., 36.

25. Ibid., 39–40.

26. Ibid., 40.
27. Ibid., 41.
28. Ibid., 41–42.

Appendix 3

1. Henning Fenger, *Kierkegaard, the Myths and Their Origins: Studies in the Kierkegaardian Papers and Letters*, trans. George C. Schoolfield (New Haven: Yale University Press, 1980), xii.

2. Ibid., xiii. In view of this he wrote: "I frankly confess that I am unable to follow Kierkegaard as he leaps out over a sea 70,000 fathoms deep—I am glad if I can survive the yard-and-a-half which was the depth of Soborg Lake in 1835" (vi).

3. His room had to be at a certain temperature at all times. In his diary, the word "cool" was always associated with anything beautiful and attractive. The curtains were always shut. He always walked on the shady side. At Rosenborg Street, he was worried by the smell from the tannery in the yard. At 35 North Street, he was disturbed by the reflection of the sun on the neighbor's window and the barking of a dog. At his last house, he complained that it was too dark and attributed the illness that led to his death to this darkness. He was sickly fearful of fire and always had a bowl of water standing ready whenever he lit his cigar. Johannes Hohlenberg, *Søren Kierkegaard* (London: Routledge & Kegan Paul, 1940), 146–47. According to Josiah Thompson, not a detail was neglected in constructing an environment perfectly suited his wishes. Fenger, *Kierkegaard*, 121–23.

4. The combination of dysthymia and major depression is called "double depression." Alan Stoudemire, *Clinical Psychiatry for Medical Students* (Philadelphia: Lippincott, 1990), 162.

5. Lowrie, *A Short Life of Kierkegaard* (Princeton, NJ: Princeton University Press, 1942), 37; and Fenger, *Kierkegaard*, 67.

6. *DSM-IV* states (p. 432): "The disturbance lasts for a minimum of 2 days and a maximum of 4 weeks and occurs within 4 weeks of the traumatic event." In explaining differential diagnosis, *DSM-IV* states on p. 431: "By definition, a diagnosis of Acute Stress Disorder is appropriate only for symptoms that occur within 1 month of the extreme stressor. . . . For individuals with the diagnosis of Acute Stress Disorder whose symptoms persist for longer than 1 month, the diagnosis of Posttraumatic Stress Disorder should be considered." My reason for not classifying Kierkegaard under posttraumatic disorder is that there is nothing in the criteria that can account for his experiences of derealization, fear of losing control, fear of going crazy, and feeling on the verge.

7. Differing opinions on this issue of fear have resulted in suggestions such as tuberculosis (fear of sunlight), conjunctivitis (heliophobia), and myelitis (disturbances of the sense of touch). Fenger, *Kierkegaard*, 66.

8. Ibid.

9. Ibid., 152.

10. Kierkegaard, *Journals of Kierkegaard*, 55, 86.

11. Lowrie, *Short Life of Søren Kierkegaard*, 52, 72–77.

12. One of the differences between major depressive episodes and dysthymia is that dysthymia is chronic, without a clear onset, relatively persistent, and non-psychotic. Stoudemire, *Clinical Psychiatry for Medical Students*, 161.

13. Ibid., 34.
14. Ibid., 113.
15. Ibid., 157.
16. Ibid., 33.
17. Ibid., 233.
18. Ibid., 83.
19. Kierkegaard, *Journals of Kierkegaard*, 40.
20. Thompson, *Kierkegaard*, 83.
21. Kierkegaard, *Journals of Kierkegaard*, 50.
22. Thompson, *Kierkegaard*, 84.
23. Ibid., 122.
24. Lowrie, *Short Life of Kierkegaard*, 98.

Bibliography

American Psychiatric Association. *Diagnostic and Statistical Manual of Mental Disorders IV*. Washington, D.C.: American Psychiatric Association, 1994.

Boisen, Anton T. *Out of the Depths: An Autobiographical Study of Mental Disorder and Religious Experience*. New York: Harper & Bros., 1960.

Bonhoeffer, Dietrich. *Ethics*. New York: Macmillan, 1965.

———. *Letters and Papers from Prison*. New York: McMillan, 1971.

Bosanquet, B. *Contemporary Philosophy*. London: MacMillan, 1921.

Bulkeley, Kelly. *Transforming Dreams: Learning Spiritual Lessons from the Dreams You Never Forget*. New York: John Wiley & Sons, 2000.

Capra, Fritjof. *The Tao of Physics*. New York: Bantam, 1983.

Cashdan, Sheldon. *Object Relations Therapy: Using the Relationship*. New York: W. W. Norton, 1988.

Cavalli, Thom F. *Alchemical Psychology: Old Recipes for Living in a New World*. New York: Putnam, 2002.

Chan, Wing-Tsit. *The Source Book in Chinese Philosophy*. Princeton: Princeton University Press, 1963.

Christie, Anthony. *Chinese Mythology*. Italy: Hymlyn Publishing, 1968.

Cousin, E. H. "Models and the Future of Theology." In *The Coming Convergence of World Religions*, edited by R. E. Whitson. New York: Newman, 1971.

Cranton, Pamela Lee. "Kaddish Poem." *The Journal of Pastoral Care and Counseling* 57, no. 1 (2003): 98.

Dales, Douglas. "Celtic and Anglo-Saxon Spirituality." In *The Story of Christian Spirituality: Two Thousand Years, From East to West*, edited by Gordon Mursell. Minneapolis: Fortress Press, 2002.

Dittes, James E. *Pastoral Counseling: The Basics*. Louisville: Westminster John Knox Press, 1999.

Dourley, John P. *The Psyche as Sacrament: A Comparative Study of C. G. Jung and Paul Tillich*. Toronto: Inner City Books, 1981.

Fenger, Henning. *Kierkegaard, the Myths and Their Origins: Studies in the Kierkegaardian Papers and Letters*. New Haven: Yale University Press, 1980.

Foucault, Michel. *Mental Illness and Psychology*. Berkeley: University of California Press, 1962.

Fryback, Patricia, and Bonita Reinert. "Spirituality and People with Potentially Fatal Diagnoses." *Nursing Forum* 34, no. 1 (1999): 20.

Graham, Jory. *In the Company of Others: Understanding the Human Needs of Cancer Patients*. New York: Harcourt Brace Jovanovich, 1982.

Hacked, Sergei. "The Russian Spirit." In *The Story of Christian Spirituality: Two*

Thousand Years, From East to West, edited by Gordon Mursell. Minneapolis: Fortress Press, 2002.

Harre-Mustin, Rachel T., and Jeanne Marecek. "Abnormal and Clinical Psychology: The Politics of Madness." In *Critical Psychology: An Introduction*, edited by Dennis Fox and Isaac Prilleltensky. London: Sage, 1997.

Harris, Benjamin. "Repoliticizing the History of Psychology." In *Critical Psychology: An Introduction*, edited by Dennis Fox and Isaac Prilleltensky. London: Sage, 1997.

Hedaya, Robert. *Understanding Biological Psychiatry*. New York: W. W. Norton, 1996.

Herman, Judith Lewis. *Trauma and Recovery: The Aftermath of Violence from Domestic Abuse and Political Terror*. New York: Basic Books, 1992.

Hohlenberg, Johannes. *Søren Kierkegaard*. London: Routledge & Kegan Paul, 1940.

Holmes, Kristin E. "23rd Psalm Holds Answers to Many of Life's Questions." *The Riverside Press-Enterprise*, October 25, 2005, B12.

Holt, Bradley. "Spiritualities of the Twentieth Century." In *The Story of Christian Spirituality: Two Thousand Years, From East to West*, edited by Gordon Mursell. Minneapolis: Fortress Press, 2002.

Hsu, Albert Y. *Grieving a Suicide: A Loved One's Search for Comfort, Answers and Hope*. Urbana, IL: InterVarsity Press, 2002.

James, William. *Varieties of Religious Experience*. New York: Macmillan, 1961.

Jamison, Kay R. *Touched with Fire: Manic-Depressive Illness and the Artistic Temperament*. New York: Free Press, 1996.

Jung, Carl. *Psychology and Alchemy*. Translated by R. F. C Hull. London: Routledge & Kegan Paul, 1953.

——. *Psychology and Western Religion*. Translated by R. F. C. Hull. Princeton: Princeton University Press, 1984.

Karp, David. *Speaking of Sadness: Depression, Disconnection, and the Meanings of Illness*. Oxford: Oxford University Press, 1996.

Katz, Brian P. *Myths of the World: Deities and Demons of the Far East*. New York: Metrobooks, 1995.

Kierkegaard, Søren. *The Concept of Anxiety: A Simple Psychologically Orienting Deliberation on the Dogmatic Issue of Hereditary Sin*. Edited and translated with introduction and notes by Reidar Thomte and Albert B. Anderson. Princeton: Princeton University Press, 1980.

——. *The Concept of Dread*. Translated with introduction by Walter Lowrie. Princeton: Princeton University Press, 1944.

——. *Either/Or: A Fragment of Life*. New York: Penguin Classics, 1992.

——. *Fear and Trembling* and *The Sickness Unto Death*. Translated with an introduction by Walter Lowrie. Princeton: Princeton University Press, 1954.

——. *The Journals of Kierkegaard*. Edited with an introduction by Alexander Dru. New York: Harper, 1959.

——. *Letters and Documents*. Translated by Henrik Rosenmeier. Princeton, NJ: Princeton University Press, 1978.

——. *The Point of View: Kierkegaard's Writings*, Vol 22. Edited by Howard V. Hong and Edna H. Hong. Princeton: Princeton University Press, 1998.

——. *Søren Kierkegaard's Journals and Papers*. Vol 2., edited and translated by Howard V. Hong and Edna H. Hong. Bloomington, IN: Indiana University Press, 1970.

——. *Stages on Life's Way.* Introduction by Paul Sponheim, translated by Walter Lowrie. Princeton: Princeton University Press, 1967.

Killen, Patricia O'Connell, and John de Beer. *The Art of Theological Reflection.* New York: Crossroad, 1994.

Kleinman, Arthur. "How is Culture Important for DSM-IV?" In *Culture and Psychiatric Diagnosis: A DSM-IV Perspective,* edited by Juan E. Mezzich, Arthur Kleinman, Horacio Fabrega Jr., and Delores L. Parron. Washington, D.C.: American Psychiatric Press, 1996.

Kubler-Ross, Elizabeth. *On Death and Dying: What the Dying Have to Teach Doctors, Nurses, Clergy, and Their Own Families.* New York: Collier, 1969.

Lowrie, Walter. *A Short Life: Kierkegaard.* Princeton: Princeton University Press, 1942.

Macquarrie, John. *Principles of Christian Theology.* New York: Charles Scribner's Sons, 1966.

Manning, Martha. *Undercurrents: A Life Beneath the Surface.* San Francisco: HarperSanFrancisco, 1994.

Marsella, Anthony J., Norman Sartorius, Assen Jablensky, and Fred R. Fenton. "Cross-Cultural Studies of Depressive Disorders: An Overview." In *Culture and Depression: Studies in the Anthropology and Cross-Cultural Psychiatry of Affect and Disorder,* edited by Arthur Kleinman and Byron Good. Berkeley: University of California Press, 1985.

May, Gerald. *Simply Sane: The Spirituality of Mental Health.* New York: Crossroad,1977.

Moore, Thomas. *Care of the Soul: A Guide for Cultivating Depth and Sacredness in Everyday Life.* New York: HarperPerennial, 1992.

"Mother Goddess as Kali—The Feminine Force in Indian Art" (August 2000): 7, http://www.exoticindiaart.com/kali.htm.

Mulder, Neils. *Everyday Life in Thailand: An Interpretation.* Bangkok: Duang Kamol, 1979.

Newberg, Andrew, A. Alvin, M. Baime, P. D. Mozley, and E. d'Aquili. "The Measurement of Cerebral Blood Flow During the Complex Cognitive Task of Meditation Using HMPAO-SPECT Imaging." *Journal of Nuclear Medicine,* 38 (1997): 95.

Newberg, Andrew, M. Pourdehnad, A. Alavis, and E. d'Aquili. "Cerebral Blood Flow During Meditation: Preliminary Findings and Methodological Issues." *Perceptual Motor Skills* 97 (2003): 625–30.

Newberg, Andrew, Eugene d'Aquili, and Vince Rause. *Why God Won't Go Away: Brain Science and the Biology of Belief.* New York: Ballantine, 2001.

Nietzsche, Friedrich. *Thus Spoke Zarathustra.* In *The Portable Nietzsche,* translated by Walter Kaufmann. New York: Penguin, 1954.

Nouwen, Henry. *Lifesigns: Intimacy, Fecundity, and Ecstasy in Christian Perspective.* New York: Image Books, 1966.

Oksanen, Antti. *Religious Conversion: A Meta-Analysis Study.* Sweden: Lund University Press, 1994.

Panikkar, Raimundo. *A Dwelling Place for Wisdom.* Louisville, KY: Westminster/ John Knox Press, 1993.

——. *Myth, Faith, and Hermeneutics: Cross-Cultural Studies.* New York: Paulist Press, 1979.

——. *The Silence of God: The Answer of the Buddha.* Translated by Robert Barr. New York: Orbis, 1989.

Pascal, Blaise. *Pensées*. New York: E. P. Dutton, 1958.

Perkins, Robert L., ed. *International Kierkegaard Commentary: The Concept of Anxiety*. Macon, GA: Mercer, 1985.

Radhakrishnan, S. *Indian Philosophy*. Vol. 1. Bombay: Blackie & Son, 1940, reprint, 1989.

Ramirez-Johnson, Johnny, Carlos Fayard, Carlos Garberoglio, and Clara M. Jorge Ramirez. "Is Faith an Emotion? Faith as a Meaning-Making Affective Process: An Example from Breast Cancer Patients." *American Behavioral Scientist* 45, no. 12 (August 2002): 1839–53.

Remen, Rachel Naomi. *My Grandfather's Blessings: Stories of Strength, Refuge, and Belonging*. New York: Riverhead Books, 2000.

Rumi. *The Love Poems of Rumi*. Edited by Deepak Chopra. New York: Harmony Books, 1998.

Samson, Andre, and Barbara Zerter, "The Experience of Spirituality in the Psycho-Social Adaptation of Cancer Survivors." *The Journal of Pastoral Care & Counseling* 57, no. 3 (2003): 334.

Sanford, J. A. *Dreams and Healing: A Succinct and Lively Interpretation of Dreams*. New York: Paulist Press, 1978.

Schmidt, Roger. "Tribal Religions in Historical Times." In *Patterns of Religion*, edited by Roger Schmidt et al. Belmont, CA: Wadsworth, 1999.

Silko, Leslie Marmon. *Ceremony*. New York: Penguin, 1986.

Sorajjakool, Siroj. "Getting There Without Going Anywhere: Chuang Tzu's Nothingness and Spiritual Transformation" (2003), unpublished manuscript.

———. "Thai Women's Experiences with AIDS: Perspectives on Religion and Coping." Accepted for publication, *Journal of HIV/AIDS and Social Services*, Haworth Press, 2005.

———. *Wu Wei, Negativity, and Depression: The Principle of Non-Trying in the Practice of Pastoral Care*. New York: Haworth Pastoral Press, 2001.

Sorajjakool, Siroj, and Bryn Seyle. "Theological Strategies, Constructed Meaning, and Coping with Cancer: A Qualitative Study." *Pastoral Psychology* 54, no. 2 (2005): 173–87.

Sorajjakool, Siroj, Kelvin Thompson, Leigh Aveling, and Art Earll. "Chronic Pain, Meaning, and Spirituality: A Qualitative Study of the Healing Process in Relation to the Role of Meaning Among Individuals with Chronic Pain" (accepted for publication by *The Journal of Pastoral Care & Counseling*, March 2005).

Spong, John Shelby. *A New Christianity for a New World: Why Traditional Faith Is Dying and How a New Faith Is Being Born*. San Francisco: HarperSanFrancisco, 2001.

Stoudemire, Alan. *Clinical Psychiatry for Medical Students*. Philadelphia: Lippincott, 1990.

Syrjanen, S. "In Search of Meaning and Identity: Conversion to Christianity in Pakistani Muslim Culture." *Annals of the Finnish Society of Missiology and Ecumenics* 45 (1984): 90.

Tagore, Rabindranath. *Gitanjali: A Collection of Prose Translations Made by the Author from the Original Bengali*. New York: Scribner Poetry, 1941.

Tan, Teik Beng. *Beliefs and Practices Among Malaysian Chinese Buddhists*. Kuala Lumpur: Buddhist Missionary Society, 1988.

Taylor, Elizabeth Johnston. "Spiritual Needs of Patients with Cancer and Family Caregivers." *Cancer Nursing* 26, no. 4 (2003): 265.

Taylor, Mark C. *Journeys to Selfhood: Hegel & Kierkegaard.* Los Angeles: University of California, 1980.

Thompson, Josiah. *Kierkegaard.* New York: Alfred A. Knopf, 1973.

Tillich, Paul. *The Courage to Be.* London: Fontana, 1952.

———. *Systematic Theology.* Vol. 2. London: SCM, 1957.

———. *Theology of Culture.* New York: Oxford University Press, 1959.

Ulanov, Ann. "Chaos, Consciousness, and Plenum." *Journal of Religion and Health* 39, no. 3 (2000): 208.

Ulanov, Ann and Barry Ulanov. *Religion and the Unconscious.* Philadelphia: Westminster Press, 1975.

Ullman, C. "Cognitive and Emotional Antecedents of Religious Conversion." *Journal of Personality and Social Psychology* 43, no. 1 (1982): 183–92.

Wach, J. "Universals in Religion." In *Philosophy of Religion,* edited by J. E. Smith. New York: Macmillan, 1965.

Wright, W. K. *A History of Modern Philosophy.* New York: Macmillan, 1941.

Index

acceptance, journey toward. *See* integration task
acute stress disorder, defined, 137*n*6
Adam stories, 12–13
Aesop's fable, 80, 86–87
Akan people, 17
albedo stage, alchemy process, 127–28*n*32
alchemy process, 53–54, 101, 127–28*n*32
alienation, 19–20
Amaterasu myth, 11, 124*n*3
Anandarajah, Gowri, 133*n*12
anger, 96–97
animism, Thai, 15–16
Asase Ya, 17
Ashanti myth, 17
Augustine, St., 8, 9
Aveling, Leigh, 40–41

Baader, Franz, 73
being and understanding. *See* meaning, human search for
being there, as spiritual care, 89–93, 95–98
beliefs and practices, 15–17. *See also* religion; spirituality, as quest for meaning
Bergin, Allen E., 132*n*2
Bhagavan Maharshi, 57–58
Boisen, Anton T., 56–57
Bonhoeffer, Dietrich, 45–46, 81
Bosanquet, B., 5
brain research, 9
breast cancer stories, 3, 27, 39–40
Buddha, 21, 25, 46–47, 82
Bulkeley, Kelly, 3, 4, 122*n*9

Canada, depression study, 60
cancer stories: denial's benefits, 96; faith and emotions research, 39–40; integration task, 34, 37–38, 42; searches for meaning, 3, 27–28, 122*n*12, 134*n*14
Capra, Fritjof, 51
caregiver roles, spiritual. *See* spiritual care
Care of the Soul (Moore), 90
Cashdan, Sheldon, 24
Chinese ghosts, 16–17
Christ, 44, 45, 49, 92, 109
Chuang Tzu, 82
collective shadow, 67–68
collective unconscious, 6–7, 123*n*21
community, importance of, 93–94
completion principle, 33
concupiscence, 110, 136*n*21
conflict model, mental illness, 61–68
coniunctio, 53–54, 101
conversion experience, 33–34
Corsair newspaper, 75, 131*n*30
courage, 44–45, 136*n*18
Courage to Be (Tillich), 44–45
Cousin, E. H., 6
creation stories, 10, 12–13, 135*n*1

danger, myth's role, 13–14
d'Aquili, Eugene, 9, 13–14, 17
David's story, 27
death: and courage, 136*n*18; in Sunahsepa myth, 108, 135*n*8, 136*n*16
de Beer, John, 4, 31
delineation process, 19
denial, 29–30, 96